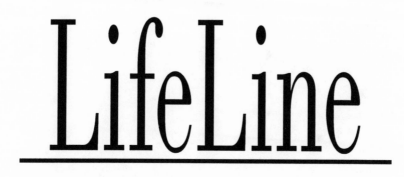

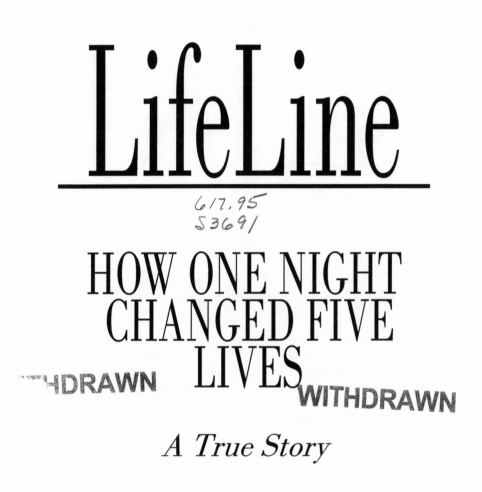

LifeLine

HOW ONE NIGHT CHANGED FIVE LIVES

A True Story

Mary Zimmeth Schomaker

New Horizon Press
Far Hills, NJ

Requests for permission should be addressed to:
New Horizon Press
P.O. Box 669
Far Hills, NJ 07931

Schomaker, Mary Zimmeth
        LifeLine: How One Night Changed Five Lives

Library of Congress Catalog Card Number: Pending

ISBN: 0-88282-135-0

New Horizon Press

Manufactured in the U.S.A.

2000 1999 1998 1997 1996 / 5 4 3 2 1

To all donor families for their courageous generosity;

To all recipients who keep the trust of their new gifts of life;

To Elizabeth, whose uncommon goodness made this story possible;

And, to Jack and the Four, whose love is their own unique gift of life to me and to one another.

—M.Z.S.

Uniform Anatomical Gift Act Donor Form

Please type or print. Complete lines 1 through 18.

1. Social Security # _____

2. Date of Birth _____

3. Donor's full name _____

4. Mailing Address _____

5. City _____ 6. State _____ 7. Zip Code _____

8. Donor's next of kin (name) _____ 9. Relationship to donor _____

10. Street Address of next of kin _____

11. City _____ 12. State _____ 13. Zip code _____

In the hope that I may help others, I hereby make this anatomical gift, if medically acceptable, to take effect upon my death. The words and marks below indicate my desires.

14. I Give
        a. ☐ any needed organs and tissue.
        b. ☐ only the following organs or tissue: _____

_____

THE LIVING BANK
P.O. Box 6725
Houston, TX 77265
National 24-Hour Number
1-800-528 2971

15. Donor signature _____

16. First Witness's _____

17. Second Witness's _____

18. Date Signed _____

Contents

Acknowledgments

It is not possible to name all those who contributed to my research for this book. Medical confidentiality precludes individual recognition.

I am, however, deeply grateful to all who shared so generously with the intimate memories of their long vigils.

This book could not have been done without the input of the professionals who work tirelessly in this sometimes disappointing, often frustrating, but always worthwhile struggle to save lives through organ transplantation. I am particularly indebted to LifeSource, the Upper Midwest Organ Procurement Organization; the Minnesota transplant centers; and LifeGift Organ Donation Center and The Texas Medical Center, both of Houston, Texas.

꙳

A very special note of thanks to Richard Ratzan, MD for his medical "proofreading."

Author's Note

This is the actual experience of a real person, Donald Mills. The personalities, events, actions, and conversations portrayed within the story have been reconstructed from extensive interviews and research, utilizing hospital documents, letters, personal papers, and the memories of the participants. In an effort to safeguard the privacy of certain individuals, I have changed all names except that of the donor, Donald Mills, and in some cases, altered otherwise identifying characteristics. The names of the medical facilities have also been changed. Events involving the characters happened as described; only minor details have been altered.

Prologue

COLLISION COURSE

6:15 P.M.

He walked his bicycle the thirty or so feet from its storage site under the back porch, out to the dark alley. The ground was softer than he expected. Temperatures today had soared into the forties, the traditional January thaw in Minneapolis. Much of the surface snow was melted, leaving an exposed veneer of crunchy wet grass under foot. In the graveled alley, frozen tire ruts were obscured by new wetness and deceptive ice pockets, making navigation impossible on his lightweight wheels. He walked the bike down the half block to the street, his feet slipping and his balance nearly giving way several times.

Finally he reached the street's solid footing and hopped onto the old bike. Sometimes he liked to push off in a standing position, using several powerful thrusts to give him a jump start—as he and his friends always did back in childhood—but not at night. Especially in winter, with unseen ice slicks lying in wait. He had become cautious as the years passed. Biting his lips, he slowly built speed. Ridges of wet, dirty snow marked the trails of cars recently driven along the street. The evening was quiet except for the slush that licked at his canvas shoes.

There was hardly any traffic—everyone was already home from work. Cars parked solidly along the curbs. Too early for the hoodlums to congregate at street corners. He would see *them* on his way home, he thought, annoyance surfacing.

Along the way, houses and apartments flared lights from every window. They can't possibly be using all those rooms at one time. Foolish people, squanderers, he thought.

Only a few more blocks to his only friend Michael's house. Midway down the block he saw the next lighted corner. A four-way stop. After all these years, he knew these streets like the back of his hand. He began to coast, with both feet loosely resting on the pedals. A small van slowed as it approached the cross-street corner to his left. A right turn signal flashed as the driver stopped momentarily, then picked up speed, accelerating on the turn. A too-wide turn. Fishtailing into the wrong lane.

"Get over, idiot!" he yelled. His feet clutched the pedals, braking. Must get out of the way. Skidding. Can't stop. No place to go.

"Look out!" he screamed.

Bright lights directly focused on him. Bearing down. Coming too fast. Blinding him.

Tires screeching. Lights swallowing him.

Impact. Head, head. *Oh God, my head.*

Body seemed to fly—up, then straight down. Head slammed again.

The world was thick, black, silent.

1

EMERGENCY CALL

6:25 P.M.

"For chrissakes, you hurt him bad, man!" a passerby yelled.

The driver of the van jumped from his vehicle, dazed, a horrifying picture etched on his brain. He couldn't comprehend what had happened. He stared at the passerby, a man who had appeared from nowhere, kneeling next to a motionless body some ten feet off to the side of his van.

"I didn't see him," the driver said, a frantic chill consuming him. "It was so dark along here. He was buried in the darkness." The driver squatted beside the motionless body.

"Are you all right, fella? I just couldn't see you."

People approached the scene—some running, others moving cautiously. More voices bombarded the area.

"What happened?"

"Oh, my god! Look!"

"Is that person alive?"

"Somebody call for help," the first passerby yelled.

"I've got a phone in my van," the driver said as he jumped up. "I'll call for an ambulance."

"He might be a goner, I'm afraid." The first man remained kneeling beside the body, but looked up at the driver.

"He isn't dead. That can't be. I'm calling an ambulance."

The driver heard his own sloshing footsteps, then, more voices. A crowd had gathered behind him. He could not bear to look back at them.

"What happened? I heard a crashing noise."

"Poor guy was on a bike. That blue van slammed him head on."

Trembling, the driver pulled the van door closed behind him, but didn't secure it. They might think he was going to leave the scene. He would never do that; he just needed to muffle the crowd's voices while he tried to summon help. He tried to envision what had just happened. Holding the cellular phone in his hand, he looked out the windshield and saw his apartment building. So close. Where the hell had the man on the bicycle come from? He never saw him until the man was bouncing off the hood.

A female voice penetrated his enclosure.

"He's still breathing. I can feel his heart beat though his shirt. He needs an ambulance. Anyone getting help?"

"Yeah, the guy that hit him is calling from the van."

"Tell him to hurry." The shout ricocheted through the driver's battered senses as he quickly dialed 9-1-1.

After the call, he waited in the vehicle as long as he dared, trying to calm himself, then reluctantly emerged and moved toward the gathering.

"Anybody got a flashlight?" a man asked. The driver was too numb to respond.

"I can get one from inside." Someone quickly left the scene.

"Hurry. This guy's in bad shape."

The driver felt drawn to the side of the unmoving body and knelt beside it. It was too dark to assess the damage, but he knew it had to be bad.

"Hold on, man; help's coming," he said. "God, I'm so sorry. I just couldn't see you in the dark."

"No point talking to him. He can't hear you." The driver could not bring himself to look at the speaker.

"Maybe he can. You don't know."

"Here, I found a flashlight in my car."

The spotlight illuminated a face that barely remained a face. The driver heard the collective gasp of the onlookers. He felt his stomach retch.

"Oh, shit, get that light off his face," said the first man.

"I'm going to be sick," said another. The driver stood, gasping for air. This can't be happening, he thought.

"Is he still breathing?" a boy's voice asked from the periphery of the accumulated circle.

"Yeah, I think so." Again the first man spoke. The driver struggled for breath.

"Poor bastard. He'd be better off dead."

"Don't say that," the driver told him. "He's going to be all right. He has to be. I couldn't help this. I swear to God; I never saw him." The gathering muttered words he could not comprehend.

"Move back, please. I'm a nurse. I need to check him again. It was the voice he had heard from inside the van, telling him the man on the ground was still alive.

The crowd repositioned itself, but no one left. A woman with long chestnut brown hair placed her fingers on the side of the victim's neck. More accustomed to the darkness now, the driver watched as she closed her eyes to better concentrate.

Finally, she nodded her head.

"He's still alive. But he needs medical attention fast."

"Listen! Sirens." Everyone remained silent and motionless as the sound drew closer.

"It's the cops," someone muttered.

"Damn! We need an ambulance," the nurse said.

The siren droned to a stop. Sandy-haired Patrolman Robert Johnston, on the force for six months, jumped from his car.

"Okay, everybody, move back! Off the street. That's right, back it up. We've got an ambulance on the way."

He crouched next to the body and looked at the woman who still had her fingers on the victim's neck. The bystanders moved closer to hear better.

"How's he doing?"

"Not good," she responded. The officer shook his head slowly. With arms outstretched, he spoke to the crowd.

"The ambulance will be here in a couple a' minutes, folks, and we need to have this area fully cleared out. Back to the sidewalk, everybody. That's right. Thank you very much. Back onto the sidewalk."

He returned to the site. "Okay, what happened here?"

"I did it," the driver said. "I mean, I hit him. I was coming home from work. I swear I couldn't see him. This street is too damned dark. No lights. Nothing. All of a sudden, there he was."

"Hang on," the nurse said quietly to the victim, who was stirring slightly. "I'm not going to leave you." She took his hand. "Stay with me. It won't be long. I can hear the ambulance coming. Just hang on."

Everyone else also hung on silently, waiting.

6:45 P.M.

Graying Police Sergeant Anthony Morgan and the ambulance arrived on the scene simultaneously. He looked around at the small horde that had gathered. The buzzards, he thought. Others, he noticed, were peering out of apartment windows overlooking the site.

"Is he still alive, Bobby?"

"Just barely," Johnston replied.

In the headlights of the ambulance, Morgan gave the body a cursory scan, then he and Johnston stood aside and watched as the emergency team slowly, gently moved the limp body onto a stretcher. The victim's face was battered almost beyond recognition. Morgan gagged slightly.

"Any witnesses?" he finally got out.

"Only the driver, it appears." Johnson pointed his thumb over his shoulder. "Most of these poured out when I came blaring in," he indicated the dozen or so people lining the sidewalk on the open side of the street "Several say they heard sounds of impact, but didn't see what happened. Others just followed the commotion."

"Lots of windows up there." Morgan nodded toward the apartments on both sides of the street. "Better call for assistance. Someone may have seen what happened."

He turned toward the driver, who had been facing away from the point of impact, leaning against his van. Suddenly, the man turned toward the ambulance as the attendants lifted the stretcher into their vehicle .

"I can tell you what happened," the driver said, shaking his head in obvious disbelief and rubbing his trembling hands against the sleeves of his jacket. "I didn't see him. I swear to God, I just didn't see him until . . ." He looked bewildered and chilled to the bone, in spite of the warm evening temperature.

"Why don't you go over to my car, sir?" Morgan said, pointing to the unmarked vehicle with a flashing light cupped to the top. "It should still be warm in there. I'll be with you in few minutes."

The man nodded and shuffled toward the car.

"Alcohol?" Morgan asked.

"No smell," said Johnston. "Just coming home from work, I'd guess. Seems coherent—considering."

"Let's do a breathalyzer, just for the record."

Johnston nodded, then shined his flashlight around the area where the body had been lying.

"Any ID?" Morgan asked.

"Nothing at all. Not even a tissue in a pocket. All I found were pieces of what must have been his glasses." He handed the pieces wrapped in a sheet of white paper to the sergeant, then slowly spread the light over the general area. "Probably a vagrant. Pretty shabby clothes—tattered canvas shoes on a sloppy night like this." He paused for a moment. "But he wasn't carrying anything with him—you know, a bag of clothes or aluminum cans, or whatever the homeless cart around all the time. They don't usually leave their stuff out of their sight, especially after dark."

Morgan took Johnston's flashlight and crouched to study the road surface.

"The driver turned here," Johnston pointed. "This set of tracks. He cut it too wide. I'm sure he didn't see the bicycle, but he swung too damned fast and far into the left lane. The skid marks start way over here."

Morgan returned with the flashlight, directing it to the point of impact, then made a wider arc of light. He caught sight of a book shoved against the curb and bent down to pick it up. *Religions of the World in the 19th Century*, he read, then looked inside the back cover, discovering a stamped pocket. "Public Library—due on Friday. Whose book do you suppose this is?" he asked.

"I didn't notice it before," Johnston said. "Could be the victim's, I guess."

Morgan leafed through the thick volume, occasionally holding the book up to his cheek. "There's a book mark in the middle. Seems to cut out the homeless theory. Call downtown. The main library is still open. They should have a name and an address.

"And take your car around to the other end of the street, Bobby. Cut off traffic until we're done here."

7:15 P.M.

Sergeant Morgan watched the ambulance pull away, then ambled toward his car, and the waiting perpetrator. Hell, he thought, this poor guy's no perp. He was just at the wrong place at the wrong time.

He paused briefly before opening the car door. He had almost made it through a twelve-hour shift before this happened. He'd been building up comp time to allow him a long weekend, but he didn't need overtime tonight. The shift had been long enough as it was. He looked at the luminous dial on his watch.

There goes dinner with my wife—again. No wonder she hates my job.

2

CODE BLUE

7:30 P.M.

A break in the Emergency Room traffic gave Dr. Tom Hartung a few minutes for a cup of coffee in the Metropolitan General Hospital staff lounge. Someone must have recently brewed this stuff, he thought, swallowing a large mouthful. It actually tasted good.

His pleasure was short-lived. A loud voice broke the quiet of the lounge.

"Incoming bicycle-van impact victim with severe head trauma."

"Okay. I'll be there." Hartung reached into a bin for a clean gown to cover his surgical uniform, tied a cap on his head, and positioned a fresh face mask for ready use—all the while gulping down the contents of his styrofoam cup. A rare good coffee was hard to part with.

A half dozen nursing and respiratory people had swarmed around the victim's cart, continuing the forward thrust and taking over the life-saving procedures from the ambulance attendants.

Tom stood beside the entrance to Operating Room One, which had just become available, and listened to the litany of medical observations from the ambulance crew. Becky, Hartung's chief surgical nurse, directed the rushing team into place. The patient was quickly transferred to an OR table.

"Do we have ID on this man, and is someone handling notification of the family?"

"Negative on both, Tom. Not even a scrap of paper on him. Sorry. But the police are working on it," Becky replied.

Hartung took a deep breath and released a long sigh. He didn't like not knowing who the patient was, or having a family to authorize surgery. But there was no time to worry about that now.

His patient had a severe head trauma. A large ventilator mask covered what was left of the nose and mouth, but his breathing was actually being sustained by a young intern, everyone called Smitty, who had immediately taken over the ambulance attendant's "bagging" procedure—pumping air manually under the mask into what appeared to be a mouth. Good reflexes, thought Hartung, watching the intern's quick response. An electrocardiogram monitor, which nurses promptly attached, indicated that the heart was still beating.

"Can we get into his mouth?" Hartung asked.

"Difficult." Smitty reported. "Not much going in."

"Pull his jaw forward and get his tongue out of the way if you can," Hartung ordered.

The intern lifted the mask further and put his fingers into the mouth. "Not opening."

"All right, his panfacial fractures have blocked everything. Let's trach him before he goes cyanotic."

Quickly but precisely, Hartung made the neck incision, and a respiratory technician, who had just arrived, inserted the tube that would connect to a ventilator and force oxygen into the lungs. One fire put out, Hartung thought. Many more to go.

"There's a lot of blood coming from some place in there," Smitty responded, looking at his red-drenched, gloved hand which he had just removed from the patient's mouth.

"We'll get to it as soon as we can," Hartung nodded.

The victim's clothing was being cut away and his body cleaned for observation. Toward the head of the table, a radiology technician was beginning a scan of the head, then downward, watching for specific areas of injuries. Lines—plastic tubing for intravenous glucose and saline solutions— were being attached, along with a urinary catheter. His blood had been quickly cross-matched for transfusions, which were now running full speed.

Hartung focussed on the patient's chest. Breathing had been restored to normal. The heart monitor reported uneven, but continuing, heart beats. There were no indications of chest injury or major accumulations of blood. However, every orifice of the head was emitting blood.

He sighed heavily. This would be a long night. The patient would either survive or die. It was much too early to know which.

3

A LONG NIGHT

7:20 P.M.

Rudy Popovich was dozing. His wife, Jan, sitting next to his hospital bed, stirred, stretched wearily and ran a damp hand across her brow. The air in the room had become stifling, dead. The heating unit under the window radiated its hot, thirsty breath hour after hour, drying her eyes, her throat and nasal passages, and flaking her skin. Looking out the window, she was surprised to see that day had turned into night. What she really needed, she thought, was a moment's respite from Rudy's struggle to breathe. It was always a relief when his ventilator was turned on. But the sound of each gasp of the machine forced Jan to regulate her own breath in sync.

She got up and made her way to the small waiting room at the far end of the corridor. It was empty. She was thankful. Large windows looked out on three sides of the hospital environs. A large lamp, with a dim bulb, shone on a table between two couches, its reflection glaring onto every window. She walked over to the lamp and turned it off. The world outside was submerged in darkness and camouflaged by snow. Returning from the motel this afternoon, after a much needed shower and clean clothing, she had thought the snow much lighter.

The wind howled so loudly it could be heard inside the room. She shivered. It was strong and mean off Lake Superior, driving snow into drifting sculptures, encasing bushes and trees—and even cars in the hospital parking lot. Thank goodness she had left their car in the motel's underground parking garage and taken the bus back to the hospital, she thought. Even then, the bus had difficulty slithering up the steep Duluth hills. She didn't know when she'd be able to leave the hospital again. Rudy seemed to be slipping downward.

She thought about the possibility of a donor heart, but she hated thinking of it. Someone else's heart. Someone else's death. Yet she also knew they were coming down to the wire in the race for Rudy's life and Rudy was losing.

❧

Their family physician, Dr. Harmon, had suspected cardiomyopathy after looking at a ream of test results. "Need to see a specialist," he said. The closest ones were in Duluth, two hours southeast of the small Iron Range community where they, and Jerry Harmon, had lived all their lives. That was eight years ago.

The specialist, Dr. Anderson, had been somber as he gave Rudy the results of four days' hospital tests.

"Dr. Harmon's diagnosis was correct. Progressive, degenerative." The words didn't mean anything to Jan. Prescription medications would ease, slow-down, relieve, he explained. But there was no mention of a cure. Somewhere in his monologue, Jan felt a stiletto prick—a vague utterance which for an instant grazed her brain and then slipped away, forgotten. Only later would Jan awaken in the middle of the night with the sharp edges of the doctor's words gnawing at her. Only then would she remember the word transplant.

But the specialist had been reassuring. Treatment would quickly make Rudy more comfortable. He would send a full report back to Dr. Harmon, along with prescribed treatment for future "episodes." After their return home, Dr. Harmon called and asked if they had any questions.

Questions? They didn't know what needed to be asked.

"Would you like to come by after hours some day when I can talk with you?"

Rudy was uninterested. He was, as promised, feeling much better. Jan pushed him into Dr. Harmon's office that same afternoon. As gently as possible, and in language they could understand, Dr. Harmon gave them the frightening news: the walls of Rudy's heart were thickening—cause unknown. The heart was slowing down, and would continue to slow in spite of intermittent periods of apparent improvement. Progressive, degenerative—those words again. But now they had meaning— terrible, specific meaning.

Rudy took the news just as he took all bad news. He stopped listening as soon as the words triggered his danger alarm and shifted his mind onto something less menacing. Jan always recognized that expression on his face. Dr. Harmon finished his explanation, folded his hands on his desk, and followed with his standard doctor/patient rite.

"*Now*, do you have any further questions?"

She looked at Rudy. He, too, had noted this moment of the ritual. He smiled, eyebrows slightly raised, and shook his head, obviously relieved the meeting would soon be over—as long as no one asked any questions. Jerry Harmon knew Rudy all too well. He had been shuffling through a file drawer looking for a pamphlet and handed it to Jan as he finished the sentence. He looked intently at both of them.

"If either of you ever has any question, just call me. Dr. Anderson has sent me complete instructions, so, if you have any problems, I can very likely take care of them right here at the hospital." He waited for a nod from both of them. "And if I have any questions, Dr. Anderson or one of his associates is just a phone call away at all times." His promises were reassuring.

Rudy refused to discuss the illness once they returned home. Jan would suffer her fears for him and cry alone. That was how he wanted it. She knew, without his saying it, that he'd want her to tell no one.

Dr. Harmon was able to handle the episodes which followed. Once or twice a year over the next few years, then more often, Rudy endured spells of increased bloating, shallow breathing, and then gasping for air—symptoms that usually responded rather quickly to oxygen and diuretics.

Until late last November.

While Rudy was being hooked up to a respirator and monitors, Jerry Harmon came to Jan in the Intensive Care waiting room. Even now, she shivered remembering his face. He'd been a friend for years. Now, he looked twice his age, ashen colored. He took Jan's hands in his.

"I've just talked to Dr. Anderson, and we agree. We won't be able to control Rudy's condition much longer. He needs to see a heart surgeon down in Minneapolis and get placed on the heart transplant list."

Jan was stunned. She struggled for words.

"But what about Dr. Anderson? He's a heart specialist, isn't he?"

"He's a cardiologist; he treats diseases of the heart. But Rudy's heart is now beyond repair, and Duluth doesn't have an organ transplant program. Only the Twin Cities and Rochester have those facilities."

Two days later, when Rudy was stabilized, Jan insisted they go to Duluth to see Anderson. After a cursory look at the charts, Dr. Anderson concurred.

"Rudy has to have a new heart," he said.

The doctor offered to arrange a flight to Minneapolis, with a portable tank of oxygen for Rudy's comfort. Jan was certain Rudy would never agree to fly. He was terrified of airplanes.

Rudy, however, raised no objections to the trip, nodding his agreement to the plan.

Dr. Jonah Dolan, the heart transplant specialist to whom Rudy was recommended, and his team came to Rudy's room at five o'clock.

"Well, Mr. Popovich, everything points to your readiness for a heart transplant." The younger members of the team smiled in approval. "So you will be going on a waiting list, and we will work to get you into top condition for your surgery."

Rudy closed his eyes again, leaving Jan to ask questions. And the only one she could think of was, "When will that happen?"

"I can't really tell you that. I think you've met Macrae; she will be your liaison and will actually enter your husband's name into the computer. She'll also keep track of your listing. We doctors hear from the coordinators when we are to show up for action."

Jan's mind raced. She barely noticed when the mass of white-coated staff left the room.

Macrae appeared almost immediately. Then questions flew. "I won't con you," she said. "I don't know when it might happen. Right now I can tell you that you're number three on the list. But that can change. Someone more critically ill may bump you down on the list." She paused, searching for words.

"And someone on the list may die?" Jan asked.

"Exactly. But I will do everything possible to keep you stable and ready. And I'll always level with you when you ask about your position. That you can count on."

"Can I go home and wait?" Rudy asked.

"Ask me that in a few days. We'll need to keep an eye on you for a while. It would be easier if you lived closer. But don't get impatient. We'll just see how it goes. Okay?"

Of course it had to be okay, there was nothing else to do but wait—and pray.

The next morning, a very different Dr. Dolan entered

Rudy's room. The residents remained in the hallway, looking glum.

"We have a problem, Mr. Popovich," he began. "Before we do surgeries, we have to check insurance coverage. Your health insurance provider refuses to cover heart transplant surgery."

"No, no, that can't be right," Jan seemed to shout. She grabbed he purse, ruffling through its contents. "I brought the policy along with me. It says they cover heart operations."

"Operations, yes; transplants, no. We have run into this before with HMOs. And I'm sorry to say that without coverage, we would need a deposit of about five hundred thousand dollars."

"Five hun . . ." Jan had never thought of such a sum of money, nor could she even speak of it.

"I know this seems heartless, but if we didn't get the money for these surgeries, we would have to shut down the program. The hospital could never carry all the needy cases.

I'm terribly sorry to have to give you such bad news. Really sorry." His voice cracked slightly and he left.

Neither of them said a word for perhaps a quarter of an hour. Then Rudy spoke.

"Well, Janny, it looks like we can go home now."

With a very sad Macrae pushing Rudy's wheelchair, they arrived at the Emergency Room entrance, where an attendant hailed a cab to take them to the airport. Macrae hugged them both when the cab arrived. As she reached to embrace Jan, she slipped a card into Jan's hand.

"This has my pager number on it. Call any time you have a question or need someone to lean on. If I don't respond immediately, be assured that I will at my first opportunity."

They would have to get a lawyer. Have to get help if Rudy was to get the transplant.

ॐ

The snow was blurring the windows of the waiting room. Or perhaps it was just Jan's tears as she waited . . .

4

SHADOWS

7:30 P.M.

Roger Burrows had gone to bed as soon as he had arrived home from his dialysis session. He had been alternately nodding off to sleep, or channel-hopping, for the better part of three hours—the remote control in one hand and his new pager in the other.

He glanced out the window; darkness covered the sky. He flipped to the cable broadcast of the Celtics-Rockets game. He muted the sound. Why hadn't he gone out for basketball in high school? Of course he knew. You had to start playing in junior high to become competitive in the varsity program. Actually, he really liked football better, at least as a spectator sport, but you had to be big and brawny to play football. It was a rough sport and Roger had no yearning to be bruised and crushed every week for the glory of the alma mater. Basketball was a tall man's game. Since he and Martha were both from tall stock, maybe someday he'd have a son who'd play. Tears came again without warning. That had been happening a lot lately when he sat home alone. If only they'd started a family earlier.

They could have done it three years ago. Martha was ready, in spite of the first inkling of his kidney disease. But he'd been selfish and wanted just a "little more" in their reserve funds. Maybe he was just plain scared of the uncertainties of the future. Of course, now they'd be in a real financial bind with a young child, and Roger on disability, unable to work. And if something happened, Martha would be left alone with a baby to support.

"If something happens . . ." He'd used that phrase often, especially this past year. Martha told him she hated the phrase. It was a euphemism for "when I die," she'd said.

~

The bad stuff had actually begun the day after the New Year holiday, nearly five years ago, when Roger went in for "a little check-up"—his first in five years. Just a couple of little problems. No big deal. He thought he'd get in early, and avoid the post-holidays rush. Martha knew a lot of doctors through her pharmaceutical work, but he hadn't asked her to recommend anyone. Instead, he asked his friend, Jonathan, who was high on his own doctor.

"Great diagnostician," Jonathan assured him.

Roger hated that first sniff of disinfectant that pounced on innocent victims when they opened the door to a doctor's office. He looked around the waiting room. Nothing but sick people and old magazines.

Dr. Howard explained the difference between a check-up and a full-blown physical.

"We should do the full physical first—to have a starting point to measure against," he said. "And after that, a follow-up every couple of years, unless something particular is bothering you. In between, we can do check-ups on any specific symptoms."

Roger chose the check-up, promising he'd come back in a few months for the complete overhaul. He suspected the doctor wanted to get his Christmas bills paid off with lots of extra lab tests.

"Okay," the doctor said, "what's bothering you?" Pretty snarly, Roger noted. He thought quickly.

"I run out of steam early in the evening."

"Having trouble getting it up?" Roger felt his face flush. He wanted to lie, but, when the doctor looked at him over the top of his reading glasses, Roger nodded.

"You look bloated," Doctor Howard said. Roger was relieved when the questions turned away from the behavior of his penis. After a bit of kneading and poking at Roger's anatomy, the doctor ordered "routine" lab tests.

A week later, Dr. Howard's nurse phoned him. The doctor wanted him to come in for a follow-up visit. Martha wanted to go along with him, but he insisted this was just another stunt to improve the doctor's cash flow. The call would probably cost twice as much for two people. He'd handle it alone, thank you very much. Martha rolled her eyes upward, annoyed with his cynicism. But Roger certainly didn't want to talk to the doctor about his sex drive—or lack of it—with Martha sitting there, taking notes. Besides, they could just as well have given him the test results over the phone. However, he made the appointment for another visit.

Seated in the doctor's office, he wished Martha were with him. When he was a child, he had always resented his mother's constant tagging along, but he had always felt secure with her there. Not that he ever admitted it then—nor would he today. But his mother had known all the right questions to ask. She listened and paid attention for both of them.

Martha had often scolded him for not having an annual physical, like everyone should. She sounded like his mother. He told her that if ever he got sick, he'd see a doctor. She told him it might be too late then. Whose body was this? His, right? Besides he'd smelled enough disinfectant as a youngster to last him forever. He shouldn't have even told her about this follow-up.

Sometimes Roger asked himself why he was such a creep about protecting his male ego. In fact, Martha had asked him that very question during one of their relatively rare arguments— rare because both he and Martha avoided conflict, almost at any cost. When she'd raised the issue, he'd obviously needed to defend his ego from her accusations. But lately he'd thought about the question often. The answer, he finally had to admit, at least to himself, was that he was afraid. Afraid that if Martha ever found out what a weakling he really was, hiding behind his grand braggadocio, she'd dump him for someone with a backbone. How he loved that woman! And all that crap about his plan for their future? The structure made Roger feel in control. As long as he had it to look at, a tangible measurement, he didn't have to worry about tomorrow or next week. Only now, there no longer was a strategic blueprint to follow. He might not be alive beyond tomorrow or next year.

During his first visit to the doctor's office, Roger had responded to Dr. Howard's questions with one-syllable answers whenever possible. Like the army said, don't volunteer anything.

Now there were more questions—specific questions. Roger felt terribly vulnerable sitting on the examining table wearing only a stupid hospital gown. He didn't want to think about where these questions were leading.

"How long has your urine been cloudy?"

"I don't know. I never paid much attention."

Dr. Howard picked up Roger's leg, lowered the sock, then pressed his thumb down against the upper ankle. The white mark remained for a time afterwards. He removed both of Roger's socks.

"How long have your feet and legs been swollen?"

"Oh, this is just that extra poundage I always put on over the holidays. You know how it is—too much rich food."

"You probably did eat too much. We all did. But you're bloated from fluid retention." Roger did not like this man. His brusqueness was grating. Some bedside manner he has. Roger would have to tell Jonathan about this.

"Do you walk up any stairs at work or at home?"

It's my heart, he thought. Mother always told me I'd have a heart condition from *the big fever.* And she'd been right.

"At, home. The bedroom is upstairs." Should they build a new master suite downstairs or install an elevator?

"Having trouble with the stairs?"

"Well, a little shortness of breath. I've been planning to join a health club. I've really let myself get out of shape."

"You can hold off on the health club for now." Okay, Roger thought, I can handle that.

"I want you in the hospital—Memorial Central—for a couple of days. We need to do some more tests." Roger felt an icy chill. This was getting too serious. The doctor wrote furiously on Roger's chart. He wished Martha were here; she could read upside down, a trick she'd learned from teaching.

Roger braced himself for the heart attack, or some manifestation that one was brewing, waiting to happen.

"I guess I indicated on your questionnaire that I had rheumatic fever when I was ten."

"Yes." The doctor continued writing.

"My mother always warned me that I might have heart problems when I got older."

Dr. Howard finally finished with the chart and looked at Roger with profound seriousness.

"It's not your heart that I'm worried about—at least not immediately. You've got blood leakage in your urine, and you're spilling protein. These are kidney symptoms I don't like. And we'd better get at them or they could eventually affect your heart, too."

Roger drove home from the appointment with a fog swirling inside his head. Well, at least he had been right not to worry about his heart all these years. But this sounded equally ominous.

The biopsy confirmed Dr. Howard's suspicions: glomeru-lonephritis, a potentially deadly disease of the kidneys. A new doctor came on board, Dr. Mullin, a nephrologist or kidney specialist. Roger liked him immediately. A pleasant change from Jonathan's man. Now they were getting some place. But he would soon learn that Dr. Mullin was not a miracle worker, just a very competent and caring practitioner.

Medications were prescribed. Dietary restrictions were listed on a flier and emphasized by Dr. Mullin. Wasn't there anything he could eat? Regular appointments were scheduled at the lab and with the doctor. Finally, there were words of warning about the signals of an approaching crisis. The symptoms he had been experiencing when he initially went to Dr. Howard would get worse.

Eventually Martha got all her information at the hospital—first hand. He should have taken her along when she offered. He was thankful that she never said "I-told-you-so." Martha was a gracious winner.

Within the year, he'd been rushed to Memorial Central twice, gasping for breath. The pressure of accumulated fluids pushed him into kidney failure and congestive heart failure. Then the attacks came more frequently. Medication and diet no longer were enough; dialysis began. For three hours on alternate days, he stared at the ceiling blocks of the dialysis lab, counting the squares in hopes of falling asleep.

Gradually, sleep came easier during his treatments, as he constantly had a general sense of fatigue. The regression of his energy levels caught him by surprise at first, but now had become habitual. He no longer remembered what it was like to feel good, full of energy. Martha became alarmed. Her work enmeshed her deeply into the medical scene, and she couldn't hide her fears. He tried to make her believe he was feeling better, but that was an exhausting charade. She wanted to cut back on her job to take care of him. Her work, he told her, must go on as usual, travel and all. One of them had to hang on to the real world—and salary and health insurance. She could call home each night when she had to be away.

However, as he grew weaker, her departures became increasingly difficult for him.

"If I'm going out on the town and won't be here to answer," he had told her with his best grin, "I'll just leave a message for you on the answering machine."

She smiled and gave him a lavish, passionate kiss—one of the old kind. But there was nothing he could do but kiss her back. He hated the lack of intimacy, but he mustered up another broad smile. He enveloped her in his arms with joy.

He tried to sound nonchalant later when he told her Dr. Mullin was considering a transplant. He tried a nonchalant gesture and tone of voice that sounded tentative, nothing for certain. Her color faded. She couldn't speak. He reassured her that this was just a minor element at this point.

But it wasn't. Dr. Mullin was very serious.

Since Roger had no close family members who might donate a near-matching kidney, they'd have to rely on a cadaver donor. And, because of the minor rarity of his blood composition, matching could be a problem. So, it was expedient that he get registered on the kidney list. He hadn't bothered to tell Martha when Dr. Mullin placed him on the waiting list. It would likely be a long wait and she had ample stress already, Roger reasoned. Besides, he'd had enough of women fussing over him to last a lifetime—well, maybe not a lifetime. He was a man and could handle this himself. Couldn't he?

≈

Now, time had passed and his disease had worsened. There seemed only darkness at the end of the tunnel. As it had several times of late, the thought of suicide went through his mind. He pushed it away and tried to concentrate on the television show, but it was not good company tonight.

He wished he could remember some of the prayers his mother used to say with him so long ago.

But, like other long-ago memories he had somehow misplaced, these, too, were lost.

5

MARGARET BOND

7:35 P.M.

They still didn't know who the patient was. They only knew that his condition was critical. In addition to the obvious structure damage, a CAT Scan revealed a cerebral edema. The patient's pupils were fixed and dilated, and his eyes did not respond to light. This was Hartung's immediate concern. Bleeding like this between the skull and the brain could quickly bring irreversible brain damage to the patient. A second scan showed it to be deeper than originally thought. There was no time to waste.

As Becky sterilized and draped the patient's head, Hartung studied the scan again.

"The hemorrhage is going deeper," he said. Many of the staff were standing on their toes to see over or around others. "Progressive cerebral edema." He pointed to the center of the monitor. Heads nodded.

Tom Hartung had done hundreds of these surgeries, yet each one seemed to be different. There was no room for error when opening a skull to reach the source of the bleeding.

With a fresh gown and gloves, he was ready. He looked at the wide-eyed intern who had moved to the head of the table and nodded. As Tom made his first cut, he hoped the intern would not faint.

7:40 P.M.

She walked into the kitchen to reheat her cup of coffee. After her nephew left, she had finished the dishes, then taken a steaming cup of coffee to the living room, turned on *Wheel of Fortune* on the TV, and promptly dozed off.

Now, her nap over, Margaret waited for the coffee pot to heat. She opened the back door and poked her head out into the darkness. The air smelled sweet and clean. She heard the sounds of drippings off the eaves of the house.

Imagine, this mild in January, she thought, shaking her head. Maybe Donald's theory on global warming is right. Of course, her nephew had theories on everything. She never knew if any or all of his speculations were correct, or just more hair-brained ideas. Of course, he certainly had the intelligence to be right.

She took one last sniff of the freshness, then locked the door. She poured the hot coffee and returned to the living room carrying her cup.

If the weather continues, I can drive up to Millie's tomorrow, she thought. This was to be one of her little mini-vacations, a couple of days with her sister-in-law in New Hope, a north suburb of Minneapolis. Not much of a vacation by most people's definition, but it was enough for her. After her retirement, Margaret had traveled around the world—literally—and made numerous explorations to exotic places. Now, at ninety, she had her beautiful memories to satisfy her, along with a few days here and there spent with her few remaining relatives and friends; simple breaks in her regular routine.

Actually, Margaret had to admit, there weren't too many demands any more on her "regular routine." Church on Sunday, playing bridge once a week, grocery shopping, and monthly church circle meetings. Her single, most honored commitment, was making dinner every night for herself and Donald.

Every night they followed the same timetable. As she put the finishing touches on their meal, she would hear Donald's tread across the room overhead at exactly five-thirty, the end of the local television news. With slight nods of her head Margaret could count his footsteps down the stairs from his apartment. This performance had become routine over the years she and her nephew shared a common roof.

Next she would hear his key unlock then relock the door at the foot of the stairs. Margaret always left her door open into their joint entry hall. But Donald invariably locked his whenever he came down or went up. Foolishness. Another of his foibles. Granted, the old neighborhood wasn't safe any more. Robberies, muggings, and murders plagued this once comfortable, working-class area. But Donald had installed extra locks on the outside doors for added security. It was she who was being locked out of his quarters.

When he had moved back into the upper flat—the apartment in which he and his mother lived during his childhood—he stipulated to Margaret that he was a man now, no longer a boy. He had to have total freedom and privacy. She was not to go up to his apartment uninvited. And, in all these years, he had never invited her. It probably never occurred to him that she always had a key to the apartment.

However, Margaret prided herself on being a woman of honor, and she had never set foot on even the bottom step. When, rarely, phone calls would come for him, she would knock three times on his door, and he came down. Aside from that contact and their suppers together each evening, their paths rarely crossed. Margaret was content with this. In making dinner for

Donald each night, she maintained a ritual which she had performed with her husband Paul some forty years before. It was good having someone to cook for. One well-balanced meal every day.

And that is all Donald ever ate. One big meal a day. He had been chubby as a youngster and detested his appearance. The self-imposed diet began in high school as he forced off "baby-fat" in an effort to be like the other boys. Now, in mid-life, he still continued the practice. All these years, and the routine rarely varied.

"Not much news tonight," he had said this evening, taking his usual place at the table. This was his stock commentary on the outside world. He never asked how her day had been; she didn't expect that. Nor did he talk much about his own activities, unless he was engrossed to near obsession with some theoretical study project. Those immersions seemed trivial to Margaret compared with what he could be accomplishing. Such a waste, she sometimes thought, though she never said this aloud. He was too important to her in her life. However, it seemed so sad that he had turned his back on everything he had worked so many years to achieve. But she tried to understand. She still kept the last letter he had sent her before his return to Minneapolis, brimming with excitement and hope.

In the process of acquiring his doctorate, Donald had made a significant bio-medical breakthrough and received an official university commendation. That week he had accepted a research job at a major university medical center. But then came the brutal retribution for his passionate conscientious objection to a war almost over—but not soon enough for Donald. Without ever lifting a weapon, Donald had become a late casualty of a war he abhorred: Vietnam. He was refused employment with a federally funded research project.

The meal this evening had proceeded in silence, as usual, except for a few conversational probes.

"The snow has been melting," he announced.

"It was slushy when I drove to bridge club today." She enjoyed any break in the silence. She wished he'd ask about her card game, but knew he wouldn't.

"Weatherman says it got up to forty-five degrees this afternoon," he continued.

"That's hard to believe for this time of year. I wish this would continue through spring."

"Hardly likely—we just missed a big storm. Veered off at St. Cloud, and now it's shut down the tri-state area."

"That means more cold weather tomorrow, I suppose," she said. Donald nodded his agreement while chewing a large mouthful of beef. "Well, at least we missed the snow."

More silent chewing. Then Donald again interrupted the quiet.

"Are you going to be around tomorrow morning?"

"No, I'm going up to Millie's for a couple of days."

"Then is it all right if I use your vacuum cleaner?"

"Be my guest." It's about time you clean your place up, she thought. It had been weeks since he last requested the vacuum. Donald never took anything from her apartment without asking. She thought about suggesting he use a shovel, instead, but restrained herself and smiled at her carrots.

Margaret felt a little smug tonight. She'd been a big winner at bridge today. The brain hasn't gone soft yet, she noted to herself. Actually, she belonged to two weekly card clubs, the newly-formed Seniors Duplicated Tournament, and her old group. Together for over thirty years, the group had now dwindled in size from twelve to a scant four. So gatherings were sporadic.

Donald used to play cards, often when his uncle and aunt visited Margaret's. But he had been such a poor loser that soon no one wanted to play with him. Once, he got into such a snit at his uncle's misplaying of a card, that he jumped up and shouted obscenities at him. Margaret had often wondered about his infrequent outbursts of fury. Where did they came from? He was really gentle most of the time. He wouldn't even kill an insect. He preferred carrying them outdoors. She decided his rage had to do with his lack of mental challenge. He no longer received any recognition, nor had any opportunity to succeed. Winning at a card game became too important. She never again set up a game to include him. Since he so rarely had visitors, she supposed he had quit playing altogether.

During dinner, Donald had answered Margaret's phone when it began ringing. He had given up his own phone years ago. Only the few friends he still bothered to sustain over the years knew where and when to reach him.

"Yeah, Michael. Just eating now. I'll be leaving in, say, twenty minutes. On my bike. And I'll bring the book along." He picked up a large volume and held it in the air, as if showing it to Michael. "You're going to love it."

Michael was a friend from childhood. Margaret hadn't seen him since he and Donald were boys. In fact, she no longer remembered his last name, and she wouldn't ask. She knew only that Michael was a paraplegic because of a diving accident while in college. He lived in an apartment complex for physically challenged adults a few miles north of Margaret's home. Donald visited him every week. A compassionate deed, Margaret often noted—though Donald would have scorned the label. She had suggested inviting Michael for dinner, but Donald said the steps up from the front sidewalk were too difficult for Michael to navigate. That problem could have been circumvented easily enough, but Donald had not wanted her to see Michael and talk to him. And that was all right.

"You'll never guess what Michael and I are studying," he said, after hanging up the phone. He was right, she couldn't guess.

"We're working on comparative religions."

She felt him stalking her, waiting for a reaction. She'd learned not to fall into his trap on the matter of religion.

"I thought you were working on the solar system." She continued cutting her meat.

"We were. But when we reached the limits of our telescopes, Michael suggested we move on out to the ultimate galaxy: heaven." He paused then, watching her intently. "You know about heaven, don't you?"

"Seems like I've heard the word a time or two." Again, she refused his bait. He had renounced God, just as he relinquished the secular world when he returned from New York.

"I think Michael is hoping to re-convert me. He won't succeed, of course."

"Maybe you mislead him with your great zeal for Father Dowling mysteries on television."

"Hey, never thought of that." As usual, he had wolfed down his dinner. With a laugh, he jumped up and took his plates and silverware to the sink, rinsing them under the faucet—his daily dose of domesticity.

"I'll tell him what you said."

While she started on her applesauce, Margaret watched him shove the book under his belt and put on his coat, cap, and muffler. The coat looked ridiculous on him—at least two sizes too big. Donald was a small man—probably no more than five-foot-six. Because of her own shortness, Margaret really didn't notice his size, except when he wore these over-sized clothes. He hadn't bought anything new since he moved back, a matter about which he bragged. First, as his own things became threadbare, he wore the clothes Margaret had saved after Paul's death. They actually fit fairly well. Then, when his last uncle died, he had inherited another considerable stack of well-kept clothing. Unfortunately, his Uncle George had been six feet tall. So, Donald rolled up and turned under sleeves and trouser legs. A tight belt held the pants up. The clothes added to his eccentric look.

The jacket he was wearing was one of those greatly over-sized items. The sleeves were rolled neatly, but the shoulders

drooped absurdly. As he walked toward the door, wearing nothing on his feet but thin, white socks and worn canvas house shoes,
she wanted to caution him to wear overshoes tonight. But she
didn't. He was a middle-aged man now—though to her he'd
always be young. His skin was smooth and fair, and his blond-
brown hair receded only slightly. It had no gray to mention. His
blue eyes were bright and expressive and contributed to his
boyish look.

Margaret savored her evening's quota of caffeine—one
cup of instant coffee. No meal seemed quite complete without
this final touch. Donald constantly proclaimed caffeine as dangerous to her health. Another of his attempts to bait her into an
argument. But she always kept herself in check. Some day, however, she would remind him that she was in her nineties, and
he'd be lucky to reach that age in good health—with or without
caffeine. Of course, Margaret didn't go around telling people
her age.

Margaret smiled at a mental image of Donald as he left
tonight. For all his quirks, she was thankful to have him there—
especially now as the years crept up on her. Most women her
age—childless widows, at that—were in nursing homes or at least
a senior citizen's apartment. But Margaret wanted none of that.
She felt safe and secure in this house she'd grown up in. With
Donald under the roof, she never felt afraid.

Well, tomorrow night, he'll have to do with left-overs. I'm
going on vacation, she mused.

She looked out the front window into the darkness,
yearning for the long daylight of summer. Her diminished night
vision prevented after-dark driving. But she instructed herself
to stop complaining. She was lucky to be driving at all. Donald
often told her that, one of these days, the state could refuse to
give her a new license. She didn't dwell on that fact. She relished the freedom her car allowed, and would for as long as she
could still drive.

LifeLine

After finishing in the kitchen, Margaret settled into her television chair to watch *Unsolved Mysteries* while she worked on the crossword puzzle from the morning's paper.

6

ALICIA AND PATTY

7:45 P.M.

"Mommy . . ."

Patty's voice dragged Alicia back from the soft womb of a wooded lakeside, her favorite summer place back home. This was the mental escape where she took her heart to hide when she could no longer stand to watch Patty slipping away from her and from life itself.

"Mommy, where will my liver come from?"

Dread lurched through Alicia. Oh, god! I'm not prepared for this question, she thought, feeling blind panic. Not now. I had an answer worked out at the beginning, weeks ago, but she never asked then. Now I've forgotten. What do I tell her?

"Well, you see, sweetheart . . ." Oh, god, no. I can't tell her that we are waiting for a child somewhere to die to give her a liver. "Remember when we talked about the donor card on the back of my driver's license?" Patty nodded slowly, almost imperceptibly. "That means if I am killed in an accident or hurt somehow . . ." This wasn't coming out right. "Then the doctors could use my liver to help some other sick person."

Totally inadequate, she chided herself. What was Patty thinking? Again the slow nod and Patty's eyes closed. She fell back to sleep.

Alicia turned away and looked out into the inner circle of the Intensive Care Unit. She pulled a rumpled tissue from her pocket and wiped her eyes and nose.

"Where will my liver come from? . . . come from? . . . come from?" Patty's words reverberated through Alicia's head, each pounding repetition demanding an answer. How could I be so unprepared for that question? Alicia continued to ask herself over and over again. I should have known it would come some time. She's too bright to think that livers are stored on a shelf somewhere and doled out to people who need them when some doctor gets "good and ready" to give the gift. The question would surely come again, Alicia told herself. She must prepare an answer. But she couldn't think of any response now.

"You look like you could use a break." David's voice startled her. She buried her face in his broad, solid chest and sobbed.

"It's all right," he said. "It's okay" He held her until her heaving shoulders were calmed.

"She asked me where her liver would come from, and I didn't have an answer."

David rolled his eyes upward and shook his head helplessly.

"What did you tell her?"

"Thank God she dozed off to sleep before I had to answer completely." Tears were coming again.

"Go out to the lounge, Alie, and relax a while," David said. "I'll hold down the fort here."

She kissed him and ran for the door, through the waiting room, and across to the women's rest room. There, finally, behind the closed door of a stall, she could let the tears drain until they went dry.

She heard the door from the lounge open. "Are you all right, Alicia?" Anna, good solid Anna. Even with the anxiety of her own son's condition, she always had concern for others.

Alicia opened her door. "Yes, I'm fine—well, not exactly fine." They both smiled at the absurdity of traditional responses. They embraced. "Thanks for caring, Anna."

"It just happens to be my turn tonight to get the soggy shoulder." Again, they both smiled. Only another mother of a gravely ill child could offer the same comfort.

"How's Chuckie doing tonight?" Alicia asked.

"Not well, but no change." She looked at her hands, and rubbed a tender hangnail.

"Sometimes I get to thinking, and I wonder if they're not going to let Chuckie have a second liver because they think we didn't take proper care of the first one."

A failed organ could happen, the doctors had told Alicia when she'd asked about Chuck's first transplant. The body can reject a donated organ. Not a thought Alicia wanted to dwell upon.

"Oh, no, Anna, they wouldn't do that."

"Yes, I know—up here," she said, pointing at her head, "but, in my heart, I'm never so sure."

"I can understand that." Alicia turned away from Anna and focused on her own reflection in the mirror. A pathetic looking creature looked back. Blotchy red nose and cheeks from all the crying. Blubbery, swollen lips.

"Does your heart send you terrible messages, too?" Anna asked.

Alicia nodded, still facing the mirror, but not seeing anything. "Worse. Patty's adopted. Both she and Eddie are. I don't usually talk about it. I guess I'm afraid people won't believe how much I love her if I didn't give birth to her." Alicia glanced at Anna's mirror image, nodding slowly, obviously waiting for more. "Sometimes my heart tells me that I was given another woman's child, and I haven't taken good enough care of her. So now God is going to take her away from me."

Compassion shone in Anna's eyes.

"But surely your mind tells you that God would not do this to Patty, no matter how you took care of her?"

"Yes, of course. But sometimes that thought is hard to hang onto when everything seems out of control. You ask 'Why my child?'" Alicia turned her face upward, determined to be done with tears. She studied the pieces of tile on the ceiling. Had the mason started at the top or the bottom? Staring at the tiles momentarily blurred the anguish. Finally she looked over her shoulder at Anna, and, again, they smiled at one another.

"Patty is very blessed," Anna said, "to have a mommy who loves her as much as you do." The gentleness of Anna's voice comforted Alicia.

"At least Patty and Chuck have different blood types, so we aren't competing for the same transplant."

"Amen," Anna said. This time they nearly laughed.

The waiting room had begun to fill. Normally only parents are allowed into the Intensive Care Unit. Exceptions were made when very critical patients might not make it through the day or night. Then, other relatives are allowed in, very briefly, one at a time. But friends and families often stopped by the waiting area throughout the day. None of her or David's family came tonight. Alicia was grateful. She loved them dearly and knew they wanted to be supportive, but their presence could be exhausting, having to assure them that everything was going "as well as could be expected." She hated that phrase, but nothing evaded the issue any better.

In the far corner of the room, Alicia saw someone she knew. Carla Perez sat alone, lost in thought. How does she do it, Alicia wondered. No husband, no family here. And this is her third time to wait. Two children already dead from the same liver disease. And now she waits and prays for a liver for little Juan. Alicia didn't want to think about Juan's blood type.

She released a deep, cleansing sigh and moved toward Carla, placing her hand on the drooped shoulder as some small show of support.

Carla looked up and smiled.

"Thank you," she said. Her voice was hushed and her eyes looked tired.

"*De nada,*" Alicia said—one of only a half dozen Spanish expressions she knew. She wished she could really talk with Carla. But a few phrases, accompanied by much pantomime, was the only bridge in their communication.

Alicia settled into the lone empty seat in the opposite corner from Carla and adjusted herself into the chair. Her head braced by adjoining walls, she hoped for a few minutes of sleep. How lucky she was to have David with her every day. His boss had told him to take all the time he needed. She suspected he would rather be at work. Well, she'd rather be elsewhere, too. But she desperately needed him here, and Patty needed them both. She felt herself drifting off.

When David placed his hand over hers, she jumped to attention. How long had she been asleep?

"Is she all right?"

"Yes. They've given her a sedative, and she's resting comfortably. We need to get you home to bed."

"No, not tonight. Why don't I stay? I've had a nap. I'll be fine."

"You have had at most an hour's sleep since the few hours you managed last night. Patty's resting and in good hands."

"But, honestly . . ."

"No buts. You need rest, and Eddie needs his mother, too."

What more could she say? She returned to Patty's ICU cubicle and leaned over to kiss her. Patty did not stir. She looked more jaundiced tonight, Alicia thought. But then, every time she walked in to see Patty she was disturbed by her yellow skin. Perhaps it was no worse than usual.

She was thankful that Maureen would be on duty tonight. Alicia always slept better when she knew her little girl was in Maureen's care.

7

A FRIEND

8:00 P.M.

Michael looked down the block again from his window. Beyond the lighted corner, he couldn't see much. What was keeping Donny? He said he'd be leaving home soon after they talked. Michael tried to remember what time he had hung up the phone. He hadn't noticed. Surely it was too long ago.

Michael was particularly anxious for Donny to arrive tonight. He was eager to see the book his friend had found yesterday at the library. He'd probably read the whole thing last night. The guy had such skills at research, and his bulldog tenacity kept him going until he found every word written on a given subject. Librarians must love a thirst like Donny's. Michael had once speculated that any woman who snagged Donny would have to be either another Ph.D. or a librarian.

At times Michael felt guilty; he had always been secretly thankful Donny had never married. With a wife, he wouldn't have the time or inclination to spend hours with a crippled friend. Donny had fallen in love once. The girl's name was Kathy.

But, in those days, Donny could compartmentalize his mind and his life. Once he began a research project, he lost himself completely.

Donny sometimes wouldn't open his mail for months at a time. Now that Michael thought about it, Donald never did anything half-heartedly except tend to the people who cared about him.

Michael had tried to warn Donny that he was going to lose Kathy. But Donny didn't take time to read his friend's letters, either. So, when he finally finished his dissertation and looked at the stack of mail on his dresser, the first one he read was Kathy's, ending their relationship. He didn't take it seriously. Donny was busy interviewing for his New York dream job. He felt he could easily win Kathy back once he had the job and could ask her to marry him.

But there was no job. The long arm of government reached out to universities using public grant monies for research, and the chief-of-staff at the medical center told Donny they could not hire a person who had been a militant anti-war activist, even though the war was now over.

So Donny said "to hell with them," and headed for home. When he eventually called Kathy, her mother told him she'd been married the week before. As far as Michael knew, Donny had never again exposed himself to the potential pain of love.

To compound Donny's tragedies, a local priest who was supposed to be a friend denounced him and others like him from the pulpit. He found Donny's view of the Vietnam war "evil and indefensible."

"This country has a responsibility," Father Berger said, "to fight for all those poor Vietnamese Catholics."

The priest's denouncement was another blow that excruciatingly wounded and distorted Donald's view of the world.

Finally, however, it was the visit of those two women about whom Donald would not talk, which struck the final blow after which Donald isolated himself from society. Michael shook his head and brought himself back to the present. "I don't like this," Michael murmured, looking at his watch for the fourth time in the past half hour. He should be here by now. Maybe he had a flat tire. He'd been telling Donny for years to junk that old bike. Actually he had a newer one, but wouldn't use it after dark, firmly believing someone would steal it. So, all winter, he used the old rattle-trap at night.

When he first came back to Minneapolis, Donald drove an old Volkswagen. Michael had once dreamed of owning a little Bug just like it, but the diving accident had ended many dreams. When another car rammed into Donny's—totaling the VW—the other driver's insurance company refused to pay Donny the replacement cost for a new car. While he fought them with nasty certified letters, his driver's license expired, along with the car license.

So Donny said "to hell with it"—again. He put the insurance money in the bank, the car up on blocks, and tore up the license renewal forms. Ever since, Donny walked, took a bus, or rode his bicycle anywhere he wanted to go.

"It's healthy exercise," Donny always said, and it certainly had been. Donny was very fit. And even in the depths of winter, nothing stopped him.

"But where can he be?" Michael murmured. Certainly nobody would rob a guy riding that pile of junk he called his "reserve wheels." And Donny would have called by now if he had turned back home.

Michael was becoming deeply concerned. He didn't want to call Donny's elderly aunt and alarm her. But, as it got later and later, his fears could not be quieted.

8:05 P.M.

"Dr. Hartung, we just got word that the police have a lead on your patient's identity. They'll get back to us as soon as they have confirmation."

"Good. Thank you." His response was mechanical. He had no time to look up and see the source of this news, or question it further. He remained focused on the task at hand, abating the pressure in his patient's brain.

8:15 P.M.

Margaret was startled by the ring of the phone.

"Oh, yes, Michael . . ." She attempted to shake her bewilderment. "No, he isn't here. I thought he'd be with you. He left here . . ." she studied her watch, "nearly two hours ago."

Margaret felt a surge of fear. He's all right, she told herself. He just changed his mind.

"Maybe he went to the library first," she said. "He could have done that, letting the time get away from him. A flat tire? Yes, Michael, you're probably right. I'm sure he's at a service station now, trying to pump air into those sieves he calls tires. And he never remembers to carry money for a pay phone."

She tried to sound confident, as much for herself as to reassure Michael. But Michael had to be right. A flat tire. The most logical explanation.

As she put down the phone, she quickly pulled it back to her ear. The line had gone dead. She had forgotten to ask Michael for his phone number. Donald surely had it upstairs, but she wouldn't go looking for it. Then it occurred to her: perhaps while she was napping, Donald had returned home and she had not heard him.

Her heart pounded as she went to his door and knocked. She heard no response. She knocked again, louder. He wasn't home.

As she returned to her chair, she found herself repeating a series of Hail Marys. Donald may have given up on God, but she never would.

8

ANOTHER HOSPITAL

8:15 P.M.

An operator's voice broke into OR One.

"Dr. Hartung, we just had a call from a police dispatcher. They think they may have ID'd your nameless patient. Found him through a library book at the site. An officer's heading out to see if he can find a next of kin."

"Good. Let's hope he finds someone quickly." Hartung said, looking at the anesthetized form before him.

"Can we move that monitor just a little? I seem to be getting some minor reflection right where I'm trying to see." The adjustment was minimal, and Hartung proceeded.

8:20 P.M.

Kate wished everyone would stop talking about the weather. Warm, spring-like, bright sun, thawing. It was as if the entire staff of the Greenwood Hospital—doctors, nurses, aides, maintenance people—were all certain that these astounding weather reports would bring about her rapid recovery. Even Bob had been caught up in the mania. No one understood that it didn't matter. Why couldn't they just leave her alone and let her get on with the inevitable? After all, it was now the only inescapable reality; her time was nearing an end. Soon all the pain and disappointments of these deadly weeks would be finished, and she would be at peace, at last.

Kate had never feared death. She'd been a young woman with a deep faith, greatly admired by those who knew her. All a sham, she had to admit. Perhaps it was simply innocence. Her faith had never been put to a test.

2❧

Kate seemed to have been born with everything: nurturing parents, a natural aptitude for scholastic brilliance. She had been stricken with juvenile diabetes, but despite the physical stresses of her condition, she had graduated college and law school, and received immediate acceptance into a top law firm. Bob's entrance into her life had led to their fairy tale romance and marriage. Despite having to watch her blood sugar levels, it was no wonder that she had expected a perfect baby to follow.

And she had gotten her wish. Though it had taken longer to get pregnant, she knew she could do it. And, when the pregnancy had finally come, she and Bob had both been ready. They had been very happy, even when she was ordered to bed. So happy. Until that moment, nearly three months ago, when everything had changed.

She was sitting in bed, listening to Bob's humming in the shower and looking at her huge, puffy feet and legs, wondering if she could get up. She was in her seventh month of pregnancy. She had expected life to get more difficult, but this didn't feel right. She had elevated her feet frequently—most of the time this past week. Still, each day the swelling grew worse. Her bouts of morning sickness, supposedly normal during the first three months, had resumed. She felt nausea now at all times of the day. She examined her tight skin; it looked sallow. Or was it just the bedroom lighting? She considered telling Bob of her concerns, but she could not pinpoint anything specific. With a first pregnancy, how could she know what was normal or abnormal? Yet a nagging uncertainty persisted. She pulled the covers over her legs as Bob came in from his shower.

"You smell good, Bobby." She relished the look of his freshly scrubbed skin, the lingering scent of soap.

"Thanks. But I didn't put on any smell-ums."

"I know." For the moment she felt demure, playful, looking at her husband. She pulled the covers nearly to her chin, hiding her belly and ballooning breasts.

He sat down on the bed beside her, smoothing her hair back from her face.

"And you, my sweet, glow with the light of motherhood."

"Where did you get that line?" she laughed.

"I don't know. I thought I made it up. It is true, you know. I like thinking of you with our baby growing inside you."

She laughed again.

"Oh, yeah. That's what this is." She pointed to the covers. "I'd forgotten I had a baby in here."

"You're wonderful, you know," he said. She felt herself blush, not knowing why.

"This has been a long and difficult ordeal since you quit work. But we only have a couple of months left. Then we'll really celebrate—all three of us."

When he leaned over to kiss her, she gave him a quick peck. Too much ardor and he might want to make love. Not a good idea tonight, when she was feeling so strange, so bloated. As he put on his pajamas, he reminded her of his breakfast meeting with a client the next day.

"I'll bring you something before I go. Maybe some cereal and coffee?"

She tried to sound casual. "We'll see. I may just catch a few extra winks." She forced a yawn.

Kate was thankful when the last good-nights and I-love-yous were whispered and the light were out. She had to think. Something was definitely wrong with her. She was sure of it.

When she heard Bob's slow, rhythmic breathing, she slipped out of bed and went to the new nursery. She eased herself into the big recliner, her hands caressing her belly. The baby moved. Perhaps she was needlessly concerned. At her appointment a couple of weeks earlier, Dr. Coslow, whom she had always called Dr. Ben, had said that everything looked fine.

"All things considered," he added. "Blood pressure a little high, not too disturbing. Keep away from salt,watch blood sugar, rest with feet up. Nothing to worry about."

Except, of course, that she was diabetic, and he hadn't wanted her ever to get pregnant. However, he had stopped mentioning it recently. Kate had known the risks of pregnancy, but she left that problem in God's hands. If God wanted her to have a baby, she would get pregnant, and then God would take care of her—and her baby.

A sense of light-headedness accosted her. She had another doctor's appointment the day after tomorrow. She would be all right until then, wouldn't she? From now on, she'd be seeing Dr. Ben more frequently.

Back in the bedroom, she arranged herself in the bed— pillows all in place to support legs, arms and baby. The exertion had left her breathless. She struggled quietly to regulate her breathing, not wanting to disturb Bob. She didn't want him rushing her off to a hospital in the middle of the night. She would be fine.

Dear God, make this all right. Please. I want this baby so much. It's too soon now. Please. Please.

The following morning Kate pretended to be sleeping, so Bob left quietly. At noon came certainty; something was seriously wrong. She tried to phone Bob. He had already left for court. She prayed again.

Please, God.

She dialed 9-1-1.

The emergency examining room at Greenwood Hospital was small, metallic, and cold. Kate shivered uncontrollably. Overhead lights hurt her eyes. The continuous examinations were torturous, and no one told her anything. Nausea crept upon her, and she called for an emesis basin, which was provided none too soon.

Finally, a resident reported that Dr. Coslow was on his way. An attendant moved her into a hospital room in the maternity wing. She dialed Bob's office again; this time she left a message.

Fifteen minutes later, Ben Coslow stuck his ruddy, kind face in the door.

"Hi, Kittie," he said. "I'll be in in a few minutes. Just want to speak to the nurses."

Tears rose to her eyes, and she breathed a heavy sigh of relief. Dr. Ben was an old friend of her parents. He had been Kate's doctor since that scary first visit when she was twelve and just starting her menstrual periods. He had tried to make it easy. After the exam, he'd pronounced her officially a woman. She liked him from then on.

"Well, Kittie. What kind of mischief have you gotten into today?" Dr. Ben's smile melted her fears. He had called her Kittie ever since that first visit. His pet name had soothed her, and the charisma still worked. After the anxiety of the past twenty-four hours, his gentleness had opened a torrent of tears. His arms took her in.

"It's all right, Kittie. Let it out." She'd felt safe at last. After various fluids were drawn by a nurse, Kate dozed off to sleep.

She drifted in and out of consciousness. Bob had been with her, holding her hand, when Dr. Ben returned a few hours later, leading a parade of white coats. Another gynecologist, a pediatrician, and a renal specialist. She couldn't catch the names.

"Katherine, I've been talking with these fine doctors about your condition," Dr. Ben said. His use of her given name frightened her.

"And we are all very concerned about you."

"What is it?" She forced out the words

"My dear, this isn't easy to tell you. You may remember that gradually increasing amounts of protein have been spilling into your urine. That is a symptom of kidney disease. You met with a nephrologist when you were, I believe . . ." he scanned her file quickly, ". . . twenty-two. That report indicated that, if the level remained constant and your diabetes could be kept under control, we needn't be too concerned. He and I agreed then that it would not be wise for you to get pregnant." He stopped, seeming to check if she was following his explanation. She couldn't look away from him for fear of seeing Bob's reactions. She had never told him precisely about the connection between diabetes and pregnancy.

"You may remember my apprehension," Dr. Ben continued, "when we determined that you were pregnant. However, your kidney function remained virtually unchanged through the past five months, and medication kept your blood pressure within marginal ranges. So I had hoped you were home free.

"Unfortunately, your last urinalysis indicated a considerable elevation of spilled protein. I'm sorry to say the lab report never came back to my office, so no one caught the rise—until I pulled your chart today and chased down the missing record.

"Well, my dear," he shook his head sadly, "I finally got those results this afternoon. They indicated the problem had worsened. The protein spillage has risen significantly. It's accompanied by soaring blood-pressure. And I know you've noticed the bloating."

He stopped to scan her chart again.

"Your creatinine clearance is now under twenty-five per cent; your red blood count is down below six, when you should be two or three times that. So you're also seriously anemic. Both of these factors indicate kidney failure. Then we add to that the symptom of nausea, weakness, and lethargy." He looked at her over the top of his glasses and she nodded.

"In effect, you are also showing classic symptom of pre-eclampsia, a kidney condition which can crop up in pregnancy, usually, as in your case, during third trimester. It has affected your blood pressure and kidneys—which were already vulnerable from the diabetes." His eyes remained on the chart.

"Kittie," he paused and said sadly. "I hate to be so brutally direct, but this is a life-threatening situation."

"And the treatment, the cure?" Bob saved her from having to ask.

"Well, the primary method of treatment is to terminate the pregnancy by inducing labor or performing a cesarean section."

Kate had wanted to scream, to pound her fists, but she finally spoke in a voice she hardly recognized as her own.

"You want to abort my baby?" Anger constricted her throat, nearly shutting off her voice. Bob tightened his grip on her hand.

The pediatrician stepped closer to her bed. "We're not going to kill your baby, Mrs. Lonsdale," he'd said, slowly, deliberately, as if she were deaf or retarded.

"A seven month fetus has a sound chance of survival," he stressed.

"This is not a 'fetus,' doctor. It is my baby. And it is not seven months yet, either."

Everyone looked at Dr. Ben, who checked the chart.

"About two weeks short."

The pediatrician spoke again.

"Mrs. Lonsdale, my specialty is neonatal infants—particularly premature babies. We really are close enough now for a safe termination of this pregnancy."

"Safe for whom?" She could still hear the defiance ringing in her voice, and the doctor seemed taken aback.

"Both you and the baby," he answered.

"It's not a matter of want-to, Kittie, this is a have-to situation," Dr. Ben said. The other doctors nodded their agreement.

"Mrs. Lonsdale," the nephrologist spoke. "Unless we terminate the pregnancy now, both you and the baby could die."

The words pummeled her spirit. Tears burned, and she could not release them.

"Is there no other treatment?" she asked the nephrologist, hearing shrill panic in her voice.

"There are some things we will begin immediately, regardless. Heavy diuretics, for a start, and a catheter to handle elimination. Also, with or without immediate delivery, we'll need to start blood transfusions, and a good cleansing with dialysis.

"You said 'regardless.' What if I choose not to deliver now?"

"Well, of course, we'd have to insert a more permanent shunt to continue dialysis. And then, along with a blood transfusion, we would start you on a hormone that works on your bone marrow to produce more red blood cells. That could stabilize your anemia."

Bob released her hand. "Doctors, may I have a few minutes alone with my wife?"

"Certainly, Bob," Dr. Coslow said. "I'll be at the desk when you're ready." He looked again at her.

"Kittie, you know I want only the best for you." He took breath for another sentence, but, instead, sighed and followed the others out the door.

Alone now, she and Bob were looking down in silence at the plain white spread over her bed covers. He had moved away from her slightly—positioning himself for battle, Kate thought.

The discussion followed predictable lines. He wanted her to agree to the doctors' judgement. She cared only about her baby.

"I won't gamble my baby's life just because I have some stupid kidney disease," she told him. "Let them give me their shots and pills, whatever, to fix the kidneys and leave my baby alone."

Bob reiterated the dangers, his voice snapping with frustration. She tried to suppress rancor, but remained adamant. Finally, they reached a fragile compromise: the two weeks until the baby reached a full seven months. Then they could reappraise the options, based on how she and the baby were doing. Perhaps, by then, they'd be over the hurdle and she could go to term. In the end she'd won; Bob's face reflected reluctant resignation.

Obviously disconcerted, Dr. Ben returned, prepared for one last attempt at changing the verdict. Chart still in hand, he studied her face for a moment, then turned to leave.

"I will notify my colleagues," he said. She knew what he wanted to say: that her life, at this point, was more important than her baby's. She was thankful he had resisted.

A battery of tubes hooking her to IV bags and machines, Kate settled in for the long haul.

She had tried to pray. But she couldn't. Dreams ripped her sleep, frightening nightmares. Always she saw a baby, and always it was out of her reach. Awake, she told herself that the medications were causing the dreams. But, much as she tried, she could never rescript those unholy visions.

Twice a day, battalions of doctors arrived at her bedside. The original four now came separately, each usually with an entourage of his own. And each had his own catalog of questions and attempted persuasions—scare tactics, she'd labeled them. .

On the sixth morning. Dr. Ben studied her chart, shaking his head over the reports. He was not pleased. She hadn't told anyone yet that the baby's movements were becoming less frequent, less vigorous. She planned to tell him then; however, Bob entered the room.

As the two men talked, Kate tried to hear what they were saying, but couldn't. They were fading away in front of her. When she came to, they were holding her arms and legs. She gagged on the tongue depressor in her mouth.

She'd had a seizure.

When she regained full consciousness, Dr. Ben spoke.

"Kittie, we've come to the wall. We cannot have you or your baby exposed to any more of this physical trauma. In the difference between pre-eclampsia and eclampsia, seizures are a pretty good indicator." She nodded and looked away.

"I'll go make the arrangements," he said. He bent down and patted her shoulder. "Don't worry, Kittie, we'll all be there with you. This is the right thing to do—for you and for your baby." She nodded, not trusting herself to speak.

Her fingernails dug deeply into Bob's hand. He did not complain. Her eyes were filled with tears as she looked at him for help.

"Bobby, I'm frightened for the baby."

"So am I," he said, sighing. "But I've also been awfully scared for you these past six days. I can't bear to see you lying here, getting worse every day. I want you to live, to grow old with me."

"With our baby?"

"Yes, of course with our baby, if that's possible."

The cesarean birth had made it quicker and easier on Kate's already weakened body. When Kate could mumble the slurred words, she asked the recovery room nurse about her baby.

"A fine, healthy girl," the nurse said, then turned away to tend another patient. The answer was so glib—or was it Kate's imagination? She fell back into sleep before she could ask again.

No one brought her daughter to her. A little too small, they told her. And she was too sick or weak to get out of bed. Just wait a few days, everyone said. And each day Kate felt less able to fight, to demand, even to move. Days passed—days hooked to the same old bags, bottles and monitors, fluids in, fluids out, blood cleansing by a dialysis. Days of pain from her incision,the dialysis shunt in her arm, and a tube in her shoulder for feeding when she was too tired to eat. Days of listening to the steady cries and yelps of the baby parades—hungry infants eager for their mothers' milk. But no infant reached for Kate, only days of pumping her full, tender breasts for someone else to feed to her baby. How long had it been? Days? Weeks? She felt too tired to ask.

Then, one day, a smiling nurse arrived.

"This lolly-gagging in bed has gone on long enough. Don't you think it's about time we go see your baby?"

Kate felt as if her heart could burst with joy. Yes, yes, it was time. The gray-haired nurse assembled Katherine's equipment onto a cart.

"Just for a few minutes, hon," she said, after settling Kate into a wheelchair. "We can't let you get too tired."

As they moved closer to the neonatal ICU, the nurse tried to prepare Kate.

"You know, darlin'," she said, an Irish lilt to her voice. "This is a very tiny baby. No rosy cheeks or big smiles yet." Kate nodded. All that mattered was that she finally could see and hold her baby, her precious Kathleen. She felt giddy with excitement—and weakness.

Kate's paraphernalia bumped and banged through the doorway into the NICU. A nurse rolled the isolette to the side of Kate's wheelchair. She gasped at the sight of this tiny, dark-skinned, fragile creature, hooked to more gear than she herself was.

"Oh god, that can't be my baby; it's my fault," she sobbed and turned away. The nurse hurried Kate back to her room and reconnected the tubes keeping her alive.

Later that day, two technicians moved Kate to the renal unit of the hospital. In the weeks that followed, the baby slowly got better, but Kate's condition worsened.

In mid-December, Dr. Coslow called Bob to meet him in Kate's room at nine in the morning. He and Kate were puzzled as they waited.

Suddenly, for the first time in weeks, she found reason to fight her way out of the lethargy she felt.

"Maybe he's going to let me go home."

"I'm afraid that can't be, sweetheart. Not yet anyhow. Maybe it's about Kathleen's release from the hospital."

They were silent then, and Kate, realizing the baby was going home without her, felt swallowed up once again. She dozed off.

Dr. Ben arrived precisely at nine, accompanied by Dr. Komaridis, a nephrologist. Dr. Ben spoke slowly and directly to his patient.

"Kate, I want to assure you that you are doing as well as can be expected. With the strain of pregnancy gone, dialysis and medications are holding you reasonably stable, but the kidney damage was severe. Dr. Komaridis believes there is no hope of getting you completely out of danger and off dialysis without a kidney transplant."

"A transplant?" Kate thought she had shouted, though in fact she heard a mere whisper. Dr. Komaridis nodded his concurrence.

"I've been talking with your parents from time to time," Dr. Ben said. "As you might imagine, they have been very concerned about you and Kathleen." She nodded. "We've tested your family, including your brothers, and, unfortunately, there is no blood match."

"This makes a transplant a bit more complicated," Dr. Komaridis added. She forced herself to return to his words. "I'm afraid it's time we put you on the waiting list for a donor kidney."

"For whose kidney?" She was almost afraid to hear the answer.

"Someone who dies, probably an accident victim." He paused. "A cadaver organ."

The words made Kate shiver.

"How long will we have to wait?" Bob asked.

"We can't predict that. Because of the baby, and the gravity of Kate's deteriorating condition, we will request that she be given priority status. But there is no way to know how long it will take to find a kidney that matches properly. We pray it will be soon."

As week after week passed, Kate felt herself spiraling through depression and remoteness, toward an end to her life. Nurses brought Kathleen to her bedside, but she refused to take her baby into her arms. She refused to bond with a child she would soon abandon and leave motherless. Better Kathleen never know her mother's touch or scent. No one could dissuade Kate—though they never stopped trying.

Christmas came and went. The multitude of holiday flowers and plants from family, friends, and associates had withered and been cast aside. Bob remained unfailingly at her side. He visited early every morning and again in the evening. She rarely spoke anymore or knew how long he stayed. But he persisted, trying to remain optimistic even as Kate grew more and more gravely ill.

The original date Kate had been due to deliver was approaching. Kathleen was strong enough to go home from the hospital. Tomorrow, someone else would carry Kathleen home to the nursery Kate had created. Bob told her about the nurses he had hired. The first one would come with him tomorrow morning to help him take Kathleen home. Kate felt shattered, and yet less agitated. No one knew when, if ever, Kate would go home. But at least Kathleen would be safe now. Nothing else really mattered to Kate anymore.

She hadn't noticed when Bob left for the night. Had he kissed her? Had she said good-bye? She couldn't remember. It didn't matter. She knew her time was very short. She would die, if not tomorrow, very soon.

9

PATTY

Now that the pressure on the brain was relieved, Tom Hartung could take a serious look at the man's face. The attending nurses had carefully cleaned away all street debris. He was still hemorrhaging seriously.

"We had to start pumping out the aspirated blood from his lungs," the anesthesiologist reported, "and we're barely keeping up."

A new person walked into OR One, dressed for surgery.

"I'm Pat Burk, Doctor, a surgical resident who has been held hostage up in general surgery." Hartung liked him immediately. "

"Welcome aboard. We can certainly use an extra pair of hands—quite literally," Hartung said.

"What can I do?" Burke asked.

"We've got to stop this bleeding. Looks like the temporal artery." Hartung continued to probe in the victim's mouth. "Yes, here it is. Put your finger right here and hold it."

As the bleeding abated, Hartung looked at the latest head scans.

"Look here," the radiologist said. "Bone splinters directly penetrating the cranial cavity."

"Well, I guess we'd better go get 'em." Pausing, Hartung straightened his back. "How're the vitals doing?"

"Heart and respiration shaky, but holding even with the suctioning. He must be a very strong man."

"And brain function?"

"EEC is erratic, but no extended flatline yet." This delivery surprised Hartung. He looked to the right, in the direction of the voice. It was the first time he'd noticed that Hank Reisman, a neurology resident, had also joined the team. Another welcome addition.

"Well, folks, what do you say? Do we continue?"

All heads nodded.

"Good. Now, one remaining request—a nice tender saxophone to soothe our patient." He looked at Becky, who understood that those who faced death often needed lightness or they couldn't handle the scene.

"Any chance of some Kenny G. tonight?" Becky's eyes crinkled. She went to the doorway and discreetly sent out the request.

9:30 P.M.

To Alicia, the evening rides home from Rochester seemed longer and more tiresome with each passing day. It had only been six weeks—but it seemed forever. At one time, this hour's journey meant she'd had a pleasant day of shopping or a nice dinner out with her husband. But all that had changed. She had no heart for shopping or "dinner out" now. Since their eight-year-old daughter Patty had been hospitalized, "dinner out" was a quick drive-through burger en route from the hospital. Alicia knew every exit ramp along the freeway, every sign. She wanted to talk with David—about anything but Patty's illness. But she couldn't think of a single thing to say. What had they talked about before her sickness?

Alicia wished she'd stayed at the hospital tonight. But she and David had agreed from the beginning that they would return home every night, if possible. Their young son Eddie needed them, too. He'd been shuttled back and forth from one neighbor or relative to the next ever since Patty had been hospitalized.

~

Patty's illness had come on too gradually for anyone to observe anything amiss. A little tiredness, perhaps, at the end of a busy day of school, dance lessons, or homework. A bit harder to rouse in the morning. But it had been Christmas vacation; children naturally get tired at this time of year—days short on light and long on excited anticipation. Patty had always been such a bright, active child—never sick, except for a mild case of mononucleosis nine months earlier. Certainly no reason to be concerned about a little tiredness. Until one significant day six weeks previously.

Alicia remembered that day so clearly. With Patty and her younger brother, she had been running errands in town. She'd stopped at an intersection to wait for the light to change and looked over at Patty. The afternoon sun had come in over Alicia's shoulder, illuminating Patty's brown ponytail and her slender, oval face. Alicia noticed that what should have been the whites of Patty's eyes were yellow. Could it be simply the glow of the late afternoon sunlight, she had wondered?

However, the jaundiced color was still there when they got home, so, the next day, she took Patty to see Dr. Lund, the pediatrician. Questions seemed routine at first, then got harder. The color of her urine? Her feces? Alicia shook her head; she didn't know. By the time your children are eight years old, you don't follow them into the bathroom. Maybe you ask them if they had a bowel movement today, and they say yes. You don't need to check on them—unless they feel hot or have a stomachache. How can a mother know all these answers?

The tall, salt-and-pepper-haired nurse took the usual blood samples, then asked Patty to produce a urine specimen. When Dr. Lund had asked Alicia about the color of Patty's urine, she hadn't known. Now, she saw it—profoundly dark.

Dr. Lund explained this was no doubt a case of hepatitis, but she wouldn't know what type until the lab work came back. She sent Patty home, recommending rest. She'd get back to them in a couple of days. Then it was the weekend, and they waited for what seemed like eternity. Weren't they supposed to go in and get shots or a prescription for the hepatitis? Alicia wondered. Was it type A or type B? Or something else? What was the difference? Why hadn't she asked more questions?

On Monday morning, Alicia brought Patty to Dr. Lund's office. The doctor found no improvement in her condition, except, she said, "The liver feels harder, tight, distended." Lund probed Patty's mid-back, trying to look reassuring, but Alicia heard the strain in her voice when she ordered a liver biopsy— "right away."

"We'll admit her as an emergency," she stated.

Alicia called David, rushed home, packed a small suitcase for Patty, and threw in a pair of her own pajamas, a robe and a toothbrush—just in case. She made arrangements for Eddie to go to a friend's house until they could get back home. Then she and David took Patty to Mercy Hospital's emergency room. They moved quickly and silently, not wanting to hear each other's thoughts. Even the words—Emergency Room—were scary. This must be bad, they both thought, and their eyes did not meet.

Finally, they settled into Patty's hospital room. A young woman doctor from Malaysia arrived to do a case history—a million questions asked in a strange accent. Hard to answer, or so it seemed. Had she been a normal baby? Had she had various ill-nesses? Did anyone in either of their families have liver disease? Alicia felt an instant of panic. They had not told Patty yet that she was adopted. She'd meant to, but there never seemed to be the right moment.

Fortunately, Patty had dozed off to sleep. Alicia whispered to the doctor, "She's adopted. We don't know."

Meanwhile, people in hospital garb continuously filled tubes with Patty's blood. David became noticeably agitated.

"We aren't getting any answers—just more people asking more questions and taking more blood samples!"

His frustration wore Alicia's nerves thin. She wanted to yell at him, but she controlled the anger.

"David, there's nothing to do but wait patiently." She directed her eyes down to Patty, who had been watching her father's nervous moves. Alicia purposefully softened her voice.

"Patty and I can manage here for a while if you want to go find a place to smoke."

She saw the relief in his face. He stroked Patty's thin, yellowed arm.

"Maybe I ought to do that, kiddo. You know what a caged animal I am when I need a smoke."

Patty smiled and nodded. "You know, Daddy, you really should quit."

David leaned down close to Patty's face.

"Tell you what, princess. You get well, and we'll talk seriously about it."

Patty's face sobered. "You always say that, Daddy. But we never do."

"Ah, but this time I've made the promise in front of your mother. You know she'll keep me straight."

Patty nodded and tried to smile. David kissed her, gave Alicia's shoulder a squeeze and left.

Patty seemed to doze off again, and Alicia walked to the

window. She watched people walking the sidewalks below. Families, she thought. Normal families like theirs had once been. She wrapped her arms around herself, fighting off a chill.

David returned, hurrying into the room—looking expectant, then crestfallen. Still nothing concrete. More tests necessary. By eight that evening, Patty had bonded with a warm, red-haired nurse, Maureen, so Alicia and David, smiling their good-byes, headed for home, filled with dread. David chain-smoked, and Alicia's mind raced. What did she need to do to prepare herself for whatever was to come?

Late the next afternoon, the doctor did the biopsy. Through a tiny incision, surgeon Addison Smith removed a small piece of Patty's liver. Tomorrow they'd certainly get answers.

But the answers were few, and left more questions. A Chinese nephrology resident came in to check Patty's incision and gave her disease a name: fulminant hepatitis.

"What is that?" Patty asked.

"Fulminant—as in fulminating," the young man said. He looked at Patty, then at her parents, and realized they were not comprehending the medical language. He knew that he should have left the opening of this Pandora's Box to the primary physician.

"It means something coming on suddenly and spreading rapidly. I am sure Dr. Smith will give you more details when he gets here."

Dr. Smith stopped by an hour later. He was annoyed that the resident had spoken to Alicia and David and warned them that it was a serious disease, but he also offered some hope. This bad thing could turn itself around.

"The liver can rejuvenate itself," he said.

David shut out everything but the final statement. But the other possibilities haunted Alicia's memory on the way home.

"This can turn itself around. The liver can rejuvenate itself," David kept repeating. Alicia tried to use David's mantra to keep her own thoughts out of range, but she experienced a sense of deep dread.

When a child is ill, a mother must steel herself for the worst to happen, the worst case scenario. Alicia felt she had to be ready—poised, prepared, so she could help her child deal with the reality of whatever news would come.

As they'd driven to the hospital this morning, Alicia had tried to ready herself. We can handle a long hospitalization, she resolved. We'll be patient, and get through this illness.

The sadness in Dr. Smith's face was palpable when he finally made rounds. After talking to Patty briefly and getting the smile she already reserved for him only, he asked David and Alicia to leave the room with him.

"We'll be right back, Patty," he promised. Her smile radiated trust.

Dr. Smith took a long breath and exhaled before starting.

"Her liver is barely working. She is in the advanced stages of liver failure." Alicia's mind raced. Okay, what's it going to be—long hospitalization? Lots of medication? A year of rest? We can handle this.

"I have shown all our results to our chief pediatric surgeon, Dr. Charles Jamison. What with Dr. Lund's data and our own, we have come to a difficult, but we feel necessary, prognosis. Patty must have a new liver. There is nothing we can do but put her on the waiting list for a liver transplant."

Nothing Alicia had done to prepare herself could ever have fortified her for this news. She struggled to breathe.

However, a few minutes later, when they told Patty, she seemed nonplussed with the verdict. Dr. Smith broke the news himself.

"Patty, we don't think you should have to take care of that sick old liver of yours. So we're going to find you a new one. A good new one that is strong and healthy." Perhaps because of the sedatives, Patty nodded. An almost-smile shone on her face.

"Tomorrow, a couple of my friends will be stopping by. One, Dr. Jamison, is very good at replacing tired, worn out livers, and the other is a very nice young lady. I know you'll like her. Her name is Meg and she wants to help get you ready for your new liver. So, will you be patient with all of us while we go see about business of finding one for you?" Again, Patty nodded, this time with a real smile. The hand of her gentle friend touched the side of her cheek, and she closed her eyes.

As he straightened up and turned to leave, he seemed to want to say something. But he couldn't. He walked straight out of the room.

Alicia felt as if someone had bashed all the air from her lungs. David stood staring at the wall, his face panicked. His hand embraced the cigarette pack in his shirt pocket as he turned to look at Alicia. She nodded to him and he left. She needed to be alone, too. She needed time. Oh god, she needed help.

Patty had drifted into sleep again, Alicia turned away. Maureen saw her and offered a shoulder.

"You need to get out of here for a while. I'll keep an eye on Patty." Alicia tried to protest.

"Go," Maureen said.

The next day Dr. Jamison seemed pleasant, but "Not as nice as Dr. Smith," Patty had announced after the surgeon left. Meg Tyler, however, scored an instant hit. She brought Patty a soft, cuddly kangaroo with little fuzzy babies in the pouch, and told her about seeing the real ones in Australia last fall when she went there for a meeting.

Only several days later did Patty ask any questions or even mentioned the transplant. Just one simple question.

"When will my new liver come, Mommy?"

"I don't know, sweetheart. But a lot of people are looking for one for you. It shouldn't be too long now."

Then Patty closed her eyes again. Was she sleeping, or just trying to shut out this little room with its sterile smells and the sounds of machines? Alicia wondered.

"What a brave little trouper you have been, right from the start." Alicia smoothed wisps of hair from around Patty's face. Patty opened her blue eyes again for just a moment, then closed them.

Yes, a lot of people are looking, Alicia thought, but will they find one in time?

10

NEWS

9:40 P.M.

Margaret sat alone in her now quiet living room, no longer able to bear the sound of the television.

She clenched her fist into a ball again. I should have gotten Michael's phone number, she scolded herself. It seemed forever since his call, and she was growing panicky. She wanted to get ready for bed; sleep might drown her apprehension. But, no, she wouldn't be able to sleep. She had to wait up tonight— even though it would annoy Donald.

She must know he was safe.

The wind outside was kicking up a storm. A tree branch rubbed against the window and startled her. Her edginess grew stronger with each new sound. Old houses always creak and groan, especially when the wind blows or the weather changes. The sounds were all familiar to Margaret. This house had been part of her life for nearly all of her ninety years. She shouldn't be afraid she told herself, but she was.

୬

Margaret and Donald's mother, Marie, were sisters and had grown up in this house. The four upstairs bedrooms and a walk-up attic well suited the family of seven children. After her marriage, she and Paul had moved frequently over their early years together, following his jobs. Marie and her husband, Maurice, had gone off to New York, where Donald had been born. The family had completely scattered.

When their mother died, their father had moved into a nearby apartment and rented out the big house. In time Margaret and Paul returned to Minneapolis and bought the house from him. Since they had no children, they remodeled the place into a duplex—just in time for the newly widowed Marie to bring her small son back to the house she still considered home. She and Donald moved into the upper apartment, and Margaret and Paul became second parents for young Donald. Life went on. Marie and Donald had been staunchly at her side when Paul died. Afterward, life went on.

During his decade of academic pursuits, Donald had been away. During those years his mother also died. Later, when Donald stomped away from the world, he came back to the one home in which he could recapture a sense of place. He set up an uncomplicated life, supported by income from a modest inheritance. Margaret had been delighted to regain her almost-son. She felt secure with him in the house, and his generous room and board payments nicely supplemented her meager income. It was a good arrangement for both of them.

❧

Fear darkened her thinking now, and her heart pounded through her head, racing. Where could he be?

It seemed that hours passed, as she sat, unmoving, in the silent house.

She flinched when the doorbell rang. Donald? No, it couldn't be. He always parked his bicycle in the back yard at night and used the outside stairs to his apartment. And he certainly had a key to the front door.

Margaret should have been afraid to open her door to the stranger she saw through the glass panel, but somehow she already knew that this tall officer with a sad, kind face would tell her the news she had already begun to suspect.

9:45 P.M.

By the time the invasive splinters had been retrieved and the artery repaired, Burk's fingers were asleep from immobility. But he good-naturedly shook his hand to restore circulations.

Tom Hartung straightened up, allowing himself a stretch to relieve the stiffness. Others followed suit, then returned their attention to the patient's face.

"Damn," Burk said, startling everyone. "I've never seen anything like this. All those splinters!"

"That, Dr. Burk, is why you're rotating through the ER trauma center."

Hartung leaned in, close to the patient, searching for other fragments of the splinter he had just removed—the piece which had been penetrating the cranial cavity.

Burk moved in closer. "But even if he lives, he isn't going to have a face."

"Have you done time in plastic surgery yet?"

"No, not yet. That's my next assignment."

"Then you will see the miracles of reconstructive surgery. Pieces of bones from elsewhere in his body, along with plastic carvings, can give him a reasonably close look-alike face."

"I've seen films—but nothing this bad was ever shown."

"Maybe they didn't want to scare you away. There aren't many facial injuries as extensive as this, but they do show up every now and then."

"Can this patient actually survive the trauma of his internal injury?" the intern asked.

"I hope so, but the odds are not great. However, my job—*our* job—is to do whatever we can to increase his chances, and prepare him to live. Whether he does is out of our hands."

11

DIFFICULT PASSAGES

9:55 P.M.

An orderly slipped into OR One and showed Becky a piece of paper. He then held it up for Hartung to read.

"Well, his name is Donald Mills."

There was a dull murmur from the others, who did not even look up, engrossed in getting ready for their next duties.

"And we have a next of kin—an aunt it seems—who should be getting here soon.

"The sooner the better," Becky said.

"Agreed," Hartung nodded, his somber gray eyes meeting hers.

10:05 P.M.

Camille raised the head of the hospital bed, trying to make Kate more alert, perhaps more alive. It was a wasted effort as far as Kate was concerned, but the kindly nurse always tried. And she never pushed too hard, or obliged Kate to talk.

"Hello, my little lady." The sincerity of the older nurse and her soft, Jamaican accent always soothed Kate. Camille had a subtle way of holding attention by just maintaining minimum eye contact, without making Kate feel she had to act cheerful or be responsive.

"Perhaps you'd like to get up and sit in your chair for just for a few minutes while I straighten your bed. There's a nice spotlight on this corner of the building, and you can see the icicles dripping off the roof."

Though Kate did not respond, the nurse was unperturbed and talked pleasantly as she tidied up Kate's night stand.

"We better enjoy this weather now, I'd say, while we can. Word is that a beastly cold wave is on its way down from the north." Her pretense of shivering caused Kate to shiver, too. They smiled at one another.

Camille lifted Kate's head and removed the pillow.

"Why don't we get you a fresh case for this? It will feel better." She hummed deep, throaty tones as she replaced the case and plumped the pillow.

"They gave me the far end of the floor today. I didn't want you to think I'd abandoned you, so I peeked in to say hello several times, but you were always asleep." She dealt firm blows to all sides of the pillow.

"Fortunately two patients checked out in late afternoon, so I asked for you to be transferred over to me."

Again she lifted Kate's head and replaced the pillow. She continued to hold her head, and began massaging her neck—a deep, but gentle manipulation of the stiff, aching muscles on either side of the upper spine, up to the base of her skull. It was that "hurt good" sensation that Bob used to create in the massages he gave her after she'd had a tense day in court. It had been so long since she felt this relaxed.

"Would you like an extra pillow to change your position just a bit tonight?" Kate shook her head slowly, and Camille resumed the straightening of the bed linens. She moved smoothly in a natural, rolling pattern as she pulled and straightened the sheets.

"Want your bed back down?" She held the control panel that regulated the positions of the bed.

"Please."

Camille seemed to anticipate just the right place to stop.

"And how does that feel?"

Kate surprised herself. "Perfect," she replied.

"Well, that was some affirmative," Camille said, mimicking surprise. Kate had to smile. This woman was remarkable. She never pressed for more than Kate had to give.

"I'm double-shifting tonight, so I hope that cold waits until after seven in the morning."

Kate wondered how Camille could endure sixteen hours on the floor. She was thankful to have her, however, whatever shift she worked.

When Camille had finished with the bedding and pulled up the final bed rail, she rested her strong, brown arms on the rail and leaned over slightly. She ran her fingers through Kate's matted hair, brushing it away from her face. Again, Kate felt herself smile.

"I want you to know, Katherine Lonsdale, that my whole church congregation is praying for you." Kate felt uncomfortable, but, finally, she forced a smile.

"And furthermore, we won't give up praying until you have that new kidney. So, just settle back and don't you worry about a thing."

Then she was gone.

Kate felt her smile fade. The shadows were blackening again. But she could not put Camille's words out of her mind. She looked toward the window. The night outside was filled with an empty blackness. She felt sad for disappointing Camille, but all she could fathom was the knowledge that she was dying. That was a fact.

10:25 P.M.

The cab driver brought Margaret directly to the hospital Emergency Room entrance. She had not often taken a cab anywhere, especially in the middle of the night. Paying the fare was confusing enough, but tipping bewildered her.

"It's okay, lady," the driver said as he reached in to the back seat to assist her out of the cab. After steadying herself, she let go of his arm, handed him what paper money she could get her hands on, and walked toward the entrance, numbed with dread.

A desk attendant took her name and went to check on Donald. Almost immediately, a tall, middle-aged man with blond-brown hair almost the color of Donald's approached her. Except for his face and hands and the fact that he also wore a knee-length white coat open down the front, he was wrapped in green fabric. He carried a large clip board.

"You're Mrs. Bond, Donald Mills's aunt?"

"Yes," she said. His voice sounded far away.

"I'm Dr. Tom Hartung." All the other noises in the huge waiting room distracted her hearing aide. She adjusted the volume. He seemed to realize she had a hearing problem and pulled a chair close in front of her and sat down.

"My name is Dr. Hartung." He repeated. "I am the doctor assigned to your nephew's case."

She nodded.

"He's in very serious condition, Mrs. Bond. We've already operated to relieve the pressure on his brain, but, I can't offer you much hope. We'll do the best we can."

She nodded repeatedly, though she couldn't begin to grasp all he was saying.

"We could not wait until you got here, so we had no choice but to begin purgery as soon as he arrived. However, I do hope I have your permission to continue."

Margaret struggled with this blast of news, but it didn't fully register. He handed her the clipboard and indicated the checked blank line on the form. She signed her name. Her hand was shaking so badly she could barely write. But he was satisfied and quickly got up and turned away, promising to let her know as soon as there was something to report.

A young nurse came toward her from the main desk with more forms.

"I'm sorry to bother you, ma'am. We need some admission information, and Dr. Hartung also needs a medical history on Mr. Mills." She spoke slowly, which Margaret appreciated.

"I don't know how much help I can be; he's only my nephew, you see."

"Are you the next of kin?" Margaret thought for an instant. She had always considered him *her* next of kin, but she would not think about that now.

"Yes, I guess I am."

The nurse handed her the clip board.

"Just do the best you can. Don't worry about anything you don't know."

Margaret stared at the forms. She wasn't thinking well tonight.

"May I bring you a cup of coffee, ma'am?"

Margaret appreciated the offer and the concern in the young woman's voice. The cup felt warm in her hands. Even bundled in her wintry coat, hat and boots, she felt chilled to her soul. She set the coffee beside her and tackled the questions on the clipboard, surprised that she remembered as much as she did about Donald's medical history. Probably because he had always seemed like a son.

One thing Margaret knew: life had given Donald too many rejections. His father had died when he was so young. Her Paul had taken over the father's role, with Donald following his every step—until that terrible day when Paul was gone, too. Also a heart attack. Then Donald's mother died. And then there was the anti-war business.

When Donald finally came home, she saw the same look in his eyes that she'd seen at all three funerals. Was it pain or anger? Perhaps both. But from that time on, Donald was different. And then the visit of those two women a short while later changed him forever. She pushed the bad memory rom her thoughts.

Often Margaret silently lamented the tremendous waste of his brilliant mind. Surely there had been other medical centers or universities that would have ignored or understood his pacifism. What medical miracles he might have worked had he continued the research already started! Why had the world been so cruel to Donald? He had always been such a good boy.

She sighed, took a sip of coffee, and looked back at the forms. One of the questions asked about medical insurance. She put down a question mark—though she knew Donald would never have "wasted" his money on insurance. But she was afraid if she told them, they wouldn't take care of him properly.

Otherwise, she decided, she'd give them all she could.

10:30 P.M.

The sound of the telephone's ringing broke Roger Burrows' dark thoughts.

"Hi, sweetheart. Your voice sounds so near." He wanted to add that he wished she were near, but he didn't.

"It's dark and gloomy here without you. How are things in Atlanta?" Roger flopped into his recliner, wrapping himself around the phone.

"Okay—but how are you?"

He heard the concern in her voice, so he summoned his light-hearted vocal chords.

"Oh, I'm sitting here with a pair of gorgeous blondes to entertain me." A lot of good even one blonde would do me, he thought. I don't even remember what sex is any more. "I'm feeling good tonight, Martha. Honest! They got the schedule messed up a little today, and I had to wait a while for my zap on the dialysis machine. So I got caught up on the *People* magazine scandals, and then took a nap during the treatment. Fit as a fiddle now."

Don't overplay your hand, idiot! He had decided beforehand there was no need to tell Martha they had to do another vein graft this morning before they could hook him up on the machine. Or that they had a hell of a time finding another usable vein. But, by the time Martha would get back home, the new incision would look like all the other slit marks scarring most of his legs and arms.

"How's the conference going?" He envied her being out there where all the operators maneuvered. "Are you ready for your presentation tomorrow?" He used to feel near paralysis the first few times he had to address audiences. That was a long time ago. "You'll do great. Take it from a pro. Just remember: think of them as being your old tenth grade biology class."

Her laughter rang through the receiver. He smiled. Yes, she remembered the pep talks she used to give him in his early days. She had suggested that he see his audience as a bunch of high school sophomores, the grade she taught then. He nearly came unglued the first time he tried it. As he stood before the audience, all he could envision was a room-full of acne-pocked faces. It stupefied him. Acne was all he could remember of being a tenth-grader.

The conversation with Martha moved along pleasantly. Yes, she'd heard it was warm today. Nice day for him to be out and around. She was solicitous and loving. But he wanted her here, now. He felt abandoned, scared. Had she felt that way back when he was the one out of town all the time on business trips? First class flights and hotels. Four-star restaurants on an expense account. That was all gone now. If she resented his travels back then, she had never mentioned it. He wouldn't either.

❧

During their second year of marriage, Martha had been approached with a good job offer. They decided that her teaching job wasn't adding enough to fund the nest-egg they wanted before starting a family. So they carefully plotted a course of action. Martha said she was quite willing to give up teaching for the twelve-month job. She was getting burned out, anyway, she said, and she could always go back when she needed a schedule that worked better for a family. She took the well-paying position in pharmaceutical marketing, a natural for her biology and chemistry degree. They made their mortgage payment from her checks, and banked the rest—interest compounded daily. And they could live comfortably on his earnings. He showed her the plan on paper. In just five years, Martha would still be in her early thirties, a safe age for a first pregnancy. And they'd have enough set aside so she could have a baby and stay home at least until the child was ready for school.

She liked his strategic plan. Well, she didn't exactly say that, but she nodded her approval. And she never said anything about *not* liking the idea.

Roger had everything so well planned. After all, he was a professional planner, working for a major consulting firm. That's what he did best—plan.

Even though her new job meant they'd both be traveling, they coordinated their schedules to have maximum home time together. That was when the plan started to fall apart. Martha soon got a promotion—director of marketing for new products. More money and more travel. So, they rationalized; with her new salary, they could reach their goal that much sooner. They also decided that, whenever possible, they would alternate their travel timetable. It was better to have one of them home while the other was gone. Empty houses were beginning to attract burglars. They were able to accommodate that schedule, and prepared lavish "honeymoon" time together when they both could be home.

Then, Roger developed a serious kidney problem. They struggled with his frequent tests and the side affects of his various medications. Some days were particularly tough, but he managed to continue his work schedule. However, the baby wasn't mentioned any more. Then came real problems. He went on dialysis, and was finally forced into emergency sick leave. Now, he was home all the time to guard the house, except for the tests and doctor appointments, and dialysis at Memorial Central's renal clinic.

❧

"Good luck tomorrow, sweetheart. You'll knock 'em dead. They'll beg you to write up their orders." He'd be damned if he was going to weaken now.

"Call me when it's over so I can give you my applause. Sure, I'll be here. Where do you think an old invalid like me would trot off to?" He laughed. Blocking out the sarcasm, he hoped. Laughter was tough with his shortness of breath. But he laughed. He was relieved when they said their good-byes.

Putting down the phone, Roger turned up the television and picked up the small, black, plastic box, sitting next to the television remote control—his pager. His link with the transplant team at the hospital. It was a symbol of failure. Dialysis was merely a stopgap measure, keeping him alive until he received a transplant—*if* he received a transplant! His antigen type was comparatively rare, they said. He wondered how such an ordinary person could have rare blood construction? Since he had no close relatives to donate a healthy kidney, it could be weeks or months—years, maybe—before a matching kidney became available. Someone with his blood type and antigen match had to die first. That thought tormented Roger.

He focused his attention on the pager. Lots of people these days carry pagers. He'd never used one when he was working. He wondered what this one sounded like. What if he didn't hear it? What if he didn't recognize the sound? What if the batteries were dead?

Listen up, old boy, let's get control here. Of course it's working properly. The hospital surely checks these things before giving them out. The young technician, Willie, said it would keep beeping until Roger returned the call to a number printed on the device. Then they would tell him how much time he had to get to the hospital.

"Before they give your new kidney to someone else. Ya' know, just like those radio give-away promotions. First caller gets a new kidney." They had both laughed. Roger enjoyed the macabre simile. Willie was okay.

"Keep it with you at all times," Willie had said. He was serious when he delivered that instruction.

Because of the graft today, they hadn't wanted to let him leave the hospital alone. But he had to get out of there, get away from that sterile white atmosphere and the antiseptic smell. He told them Martha was waiting for him downstairs and grabbed a cab to bring him home.

The middle-aged cab driver with the long, stringy, black hair was a character—a philosopher. "I'm a poet by passion," he said, "and a cab driver to support my passion." He recited some of his poetry for Roger. But what did Roger know about poetry? However, to be polite, he pretended. Or perhaps he was afraid of the silence if he didn't respond.

The stuff the guy recited sounded powerful even to Roger. One poem was about loss, about the grief of waiting for something else to replace what was lost, the fear of the unknown, aware that the unknown may be worse than the present desperation. The poem really hit Roger. Maybe he wasn't the only one in the world waiting to replace something lost, and frightened at what it might cost. Roger had always thought poets were either dead or worthless, too lazy to work. But not this one. Roger was awed by his skill in creating moods and feelings that an ordinary person could understand. When he asked Roger what he did, it was Roger who felt worthless.

"I'm a kidney specialist," Roger said facetiously.

The poet, who thought he was serious, was impressed.

The ride, however, had ended. And Roger was alone again. Of course, he could call one of their friends, or someone from work—maybe just to talk. But he'd really lost touch with everyone lately. Most people got uncomfortable around sick people, he'd discovered.

Roger didn't blame them. Look at how he was feeling now. He was uncomfortable with himself. He had lost a lot of weight, except during the bouts of bloating. Martha had bought him new slacks with elastic waist bands to fit any size. But he was still uncomfortable around friends. He hated their forced cheerfulness, and having to pretend for them that he felt great, when he was almost too tired to stand up.

There are people who can handle illness with dignity. He met lots of them at dialysis sessions. But Roger wasn't one of them. He felt like a wimp most of the time. He had always been able to avoid thinking about the negatives in life, but now he had too much time to think, and negatives were about all he found to wallow in these days. Whatever was going on inside his body terrified him, and he hated it and himself for not being able to endure it the way he thought he should.

And then the thought of suicide came back. This time it was harder to shake it off.

12

LEGAL MATTERS

10:45 P.M.

As Margaret sat stoically waiting in the lounge, the battle to save Donald Mills continued. It was all but impossible to keep up with the escalating problems that manifested themselves as Tom Hartung moved from one crisis to another.

Above their masks those around him wore looks of increasing frustration. They wanted Donald Mills to live but, despite all their efforts, he had not turned the corner. In fact, his condition was worsening.

Suddenly the patient went into a severe seizure.

"Hang on to him, everybody, we want to keep him from more extensive injuries to himself." And hang on they did. But Hartung feared his patient was about to cascade. When that happened, one after another his body systems would shut down, each triggering another factor until it arrested every function not controlled by machinery.

Tom Hartung put into effect the last desperate measures he could to halt the downward spiral.

10:50 P.M.

Jan no longer watched the storm outside, though she knew it was still there. Her eyes felt nearly swollen shut from crying. She dug into her pockets and then walked across the darkened waiting room to the lamp table, groping for the box of tissues she'd noticed earlier. She sat in the adjoining chair, wiping her eyes and blowing her nose.

Why Rudy, Lord? Why us?

She had nearly accepted the inevitability of Rudy's dying after that last trip to Minneapolis. She had stopped asking for miracles, and asked only for a peaceful closing to whatever time Rudy had left. Then came the possibility of one, unexpected miracle—a for a transplant. It was only a glimmer of hope, but surely this was a sign. God wanted Rudy to live.

২

Julie was Rudy's favorite nurse at St. Luke's. She always teased him about being a "Raincher," a name gently mocking the accent of the Slavic and Croatian people who had settled and worked for generations on the Masabe Iron Range. Julie was also a Croate, so the teasing was done and accepted lovingly.

After Dr. Dolan's terrifying announcement that Rudy's insurance was running out, Jan had walked the halls, staring straight ahead, commanding herself not to cry. She must continue to be brave *No, that was impossible.* But she would act brave for Rudy. When Julie had approached her with open arms, Jan collapsed.

In the bright, sunlit, waiting room, Julie led her to a small settee. She wrote a name and phone number on a small pad she carried in her pocket, tore off the page, and gave it to Jan. Jan stared at the writing through wet, swollen eyes, unable to read or comprehend.

"His name is Jim Crosby. He's the brother of my room-mate. Works for a small law firm here in Duluth. His father died some years ago because there was no money for a transplant operation. He's made a private crusade out of getting people money they must have to save their lives." She held Jan's hand firmly as she spoke.

"I can't make you any promises, but I know he'll want to hear about your problem."

It had been mid afternoon when Jim Crosby returned to his office from court. He looked so young. Jan was the only one in the waiting room.

"Have you had lunch yet?"

She shook her head. "I haven't been thinking much about food." His smile was warm and kind. It was as though he had always been a friend of the family.

Questions and answers were brief, asked between hurried bites into vending machine sandwiches. He gulped on a carton of milk to help push the food down.

"How bad is he?" he asked.

"Very bad. End stage, they say"

"Then we'd better get to it immediately."

He was hopeful, he said, that at least he might get a grace period for them. Jan left their health plan literature with him, and accepted his promise to get back to her the first of the week.

As she walked back to the hospital, Jan wondered what to tell Rudy. She hated to give him false hope, but she had never lied to her husband. Of course, she rationalized, this wasn't really lying—just omission. But, by the time she got back to his room, her arguments were moot. Rudy was back in Intensive Care with another episode.

Once again, Jan carried the accumulated plants and flowers out to the waiting room for others to enjoy. After selecting two vases of fresh flowers, she took them to the hospital chapel. The plants she could return to Rudy's room again when he could leave ICU, but the chapel was a proper place for fresh flowers. She would never take them back of course; it wasn't right to take flowers away from the altar. You didn't take back what you gave to the Lord.

She set the bouquets on the floor in front of the altar and slipped into a pew. There were no kneelers in this multi-use chapel. After all the years at their home parish, with its centuries of tradition, the room didn't feel like a church, although each minister, priest, and rabbi seemed to pop in on schedule to offer services of consolation to any believers who came. Yet, weren't they all there praying to the same God, asking for healing, for miracles, for courage to face the worst? She heard footsteps. A young woman in a bathrobe slid into a pew on the other side of the aisle and clasped her hands.

"Wherever two or more are gathered . . ." Jan remembered. For the moment, she felt safe, listened to, assured. Jan said her prayers silently.

Six of their children had come on Saturday. They wanted to know when the transplant could be done. She took them to the lounge and, finally, told them about the insurance company, and about Jim Crosby's feather of hope. Stunned, they clutched one another, reaching out in fear and pain, forming a cluster of love, knitting itself into an interconnected whole with Jan in its center.

"The Lord is my Shepherd," Jan prayed. Their voices soon joined hers.

Late that night she had sent them back to her motel room to sleep on the beds, chairs and floor. She spent the night on the ICU waiting room couch. By Sunday afternoon Rudy had rallied once again from the crisis. Everyone felt safer again. In the early evening the children left for home. Jan decided to wait a while longer before telling Rudy about Jim Crosby.

Monday noon the attorney arrived at Rudy's bedside. Jan nervously introduced him to Rudy.

"I haven't told him," she said. "He had another bad spell over the weekend."

"Well, in that case, Mr. Popovich, your wife and I have some good news for you." Jan had felt a surge of hope, her hands reached for Rudy's.

Jim whipped a piece of paper out of his brief case.

"This, Mr. Popovich, is a restraining order. It means your health plan must approve your being put back on the waiting list for your transplant for the next ten days. That gives us and your insurance provider time to submit further briefs: basically, the reasons we believe they should cover your transplant surgery. The insurance company, of course, will try to show why they don't have to."

Rudy stared at him, then looked at Jan, completely baffled. She was nodding vigorously.

"I'll do the best I can, Mr. Popovich. I can't promise a win if we have to go to a full court trial. But at least from now until January sixteenth you're on the list. I sure hope you people know how to pray."

After the young attorney had left, euphoria swept Rudy and Jan into a long embrace. They cried and they laughed. They had a reprieve. And that was reason for celebration. One ghost had been constrained—for ten days at least.

"Let's call the kids tonight," Jan said. They'll be so excited."

"No," Rudy said, ever the pragmatist. "There's no reason to tell them and raise their hopes. The chances are still slim that we'll get a heart in ten days."

He was right. The celebration ended. Days passed. Only a miracle could help them—another person's death.

The kids and their spouses came again the next Saturday, bringing several changes of clean clothes for Jan. It was obviously going to be a longer wait than she'd expected. Between his dozing, Rudy had been hugged and kissed by each. Jan played her role staunchly: cheerful, optimistic, everything she had to be. But her mind never lost track of the time that remained. They were well past the half-way point. Four days left.

෴

Jan walked back to the window, and stared out once again at the blustering storm. She pressed her face against the glass, trying to cool her hot, tear-wetted cheeks. She could not escape the countdown; today was Tuesday, the fifteenth. Just one more day left.

As the wind howled around the windows in front of her, dark dervishes were taking form.

10:55 P.M.

Time had stopped. Or Margaret was too confused and tired to keep track any longer. The nurse returned with a pillow and a blanket, encouraging Margaret to lie down on the waiting room couch to rest. She couldn't sleep, but stretching out was a relief. People, so many people, moved back and forth through rooms and corridors. Some moaned while being pushed in on stretchers. Others were followed by sobbing family members, frightened that their loved ones were dying. She watched a man in an electric wheel chair manipulate it through the main door. At the desk, the nurse pointed him toward Margaret, and he steered toward her. She tried to sit up.

"Please, don't get up, Mrs. Bond. I'm Michael."

He looked older than she expected. Donald appeared so much younger than his age that sometimes she tended to see him as still a boy.

"I wanted to call you, but I didn't have your phone number," she said. "I'm sorry. How did you find out?"

"When he didn't call, I began phoning the police and the hospitals. Finally, they got him on computer at the police station."

"They found me through his library card."

"Of course," he said, smiling at the revelation. "The Comparative Religions volume." The brief smile disappeared. "He said he was bringing it tonight. He's been very excited about something he found in it." Tears were forming in his eyes.

He looked back toward the desk for composure, and then at Margaret again.

"They say they don't have any information yet."

"They're operating now, but the doctor said there wasn't much hope."

"It's my fault." His anguish broke through. "If it weren't for me he wouldn't have come out tonight. Every time the streets are bad, I tell him not to use the bicycle. But, every time, I also pray he'll come anyway. The time we spend studying, arguing, digesting ideas is so important to me." His voice gave way.

"It wasn't your fault, Michael. Donald never did anything he didn't want to do. And he could have walked, you know. I gave up a long time ago worrying about him and that bike." She hoped Michael couldn't see the fib.

She watched Michael wipe his face—a handsome face. She tried to remember him as a child—the two little boys, playing together out on the back stairs. She remembered the sounds of their bounding up and down those old steps. She wanted to have them both that way again. Why did those two, dear little boys have to grow up in such a difficult world. She felt the searing tears choking her. She clutched Michael's arm. She would not cry. She would control herself now. There would be time to cry later, alone. Michael did not move until she had composed herself and was able to look at him again.

At least it is good to know that Donald has a friend like this, she thought. If only I could have known him earlier.

But that wouldn't have changed tonight, would it?

13

COLORED LIGHTS

11:00 P.M.

As Alicia and David drove in their long driveway, they noticed the colored lights blazing from inside the house.

"The Christmas tree lights are on," David said.

"Obviously," Alicia said, immediately sorry for the sarcasm.

Eddie was asleep on the family room sofa, his head resting on his grandmother's lap. The bright bulbs highlighted the nearly bald branches of the tree. Alicia stood, shaking her head at the skeleton of the once-full, old pine. Her mother had obviously been dozing as they came through the door.

She, too, looked at the tree and laughed.

"I thought we'd take it down this afternoon, but Eddie said we couldn't," she said, pointing to her grandson. "Not until Patty came home."

David took their jackets to the front closet, and Alicia leaned over to give her mother a kiss. "I know. We've wanted to talk to him about that, but we haven't had time to take the tree down anyhow."

"Well, it's a damned fire hazard now," said David, with his usual directness.

Alicia nodded and walked around to the front of the sofa, kneeling next to her mother, watching her son sleep.

"How's Patty tonight?" her mother asked. Alicia felt the pall fall over her again.

"No change. At least that's what they keep telling us. But she seems to sleep much more."

"Isn't it possible it's just the boredom of that same place? Nothing fun to do, no friends. Just the same things every day. That would make me want to sleep all the time."

"You could be right, Mom," Alicia said. "I hope you are."

But Alicia knew she was just reassuring her mother so that she wouldn't worry. Patty's condition was worsening. They all knew it.

She put one hand under Eddie's neck, and the other beneath his knees, standing him upright.

"Come on, little tiger, time for bed." Eddie awoke, startled, then grabbed his mother around the neck and clung tightly.

"It's okay, sweetheart. You must have had a bad dream." She lifted him with both arms.

"Wow, are you ever getting to be a big guy. You'll be carrying me before long." She walked slowly toward his bedroom.

"When's Patty coming home, Mommy?" he said. His voice was muffled in her shoulder.

"I don't know, baby. Just as soon as she can get her new liver."

"Is Patty gonna die?"

"No, of course not."

"Joey and Greg said she was dying. They said everybody in town is praying for her. But she's gonna die anyway."

She set him down on his bed and knelt in front of him.

"I don't care what they said, Eddie. Your sister is not going to die. I'm sure everybody is worried about Patty just as you and grandma, and all of us are. And maybe they don't understand organ transplants—how a doctor can replace a sick part of someone's body with a new, healthy part, and the person will be just fine." Eddie looked at her with a dead-serious expression.

"Eddie, have I ever lied to you about anything?" He shook his head solemnly.

"Then I tell you the truth right now; Patty is not going to die. God won't let that happen." She was astounded by the fierceness of her own voice.

"Now, do you believe me?" He nodded.

"Yes, Mommy, I do." He grabbed her neck ferociously for another hug. Then she settled him back on his bed, drawing the covers up around him.

"About the Christmas tree—"

"Mommy, you said we could keep it up until Patty came home again."

She had made the promise while Patty was home for a few days over the holidays.

They'd been able to arrange a home furlough for her over Christmas only because one of Dr. Lund's nurses offered to hook up Patty's catheter, and come by twice daily to monitor her condition. The night she came home, three days before Christmas, they decorated the tree. Patty wanted to help, but was barely able to do more than unwrap a few ornaments. She had slept on the sofa the whole week. Though she slept most of the time, the tree's lights were kept on for her anytime she woke up.

Christmas Eve had been quiet. Alicia hadn't had time to shop for the usual bazaar of delights for the kids. But life had slowed down to such a gentle pace that no one noticed. Family and friends insisted on bringing in food—even a complete Christmas dinner—along with more gifts. Their minister stopped by on Christmas day. Alicia and David were grateful for his gesture of support and his report on all the prayers being said throughout the area for Patty. She slept during his visit.

All in all, it was a lovely holiday. After opening the gifts, Alicia had remarked to David:

"The one thing different about this Christmas is that I am so relaxed!"

Patty's eyes had been closed, but she was awake.

"Maybe I'll have to pretend I'm sick over Christmas next year, too, mommy, so people will feel sorry for us, and you can be relaxed again." They had all laughed.

"Not a bad idea, kiddo," David had said.

Christmas, they all agreed, should be a day off for the nurse, but by late afternoon Patty had become increasingly lethargic. Dr. Lund came by to set up a new IV. She responded well for four days, then began a long, slow, slide downward. Dr. Lund or one of the nurses came regularly around the clock to replace IV bags and check her. It was getting harder to rouse Patty for food and medications. Her body was bloating. Urine output slowed to a very dark drip. Both Eddie and Patty were dejected when she had to return to the hospital before the New Year had arrived. In an effort to boost her spirits, Eddie promised his sister they wouldn't take the tree down until she came home again for good.

"Promise?" she asked him, and looked to her parents for confirmation. They had to agree.

Now, three weeks later, she occasionally asked about the tree, and always smiled when told it was still there. And Eddie still insisted on keeping his promise to her.

"Tell you what, Eddie," David said from the doorway, "This old tree is going to catch fire one of these days, and we won't have a house for Patty to come home to."

Eddie looked sharply at his father, then to Alicia, hoping for a reinforcement. David walked to the bed and sat on the edge.

"So, I propose we take this one down and keep all the boxes of ornaments right out in the family room. When Patty has her transplant, we'll go out to the woods behind Grandpa's farm and find the best tree he has. And we'll put it up, nice and fresh, for Patty to enjoy when she gets home."

Eddie eyed him skeptically. Again he checked out his mother. She was enormously relieved.

"Sounds great to me," she said. "Tomorrow, you can call Grandpa and tell him. On second thought, let's make that *ask* him."

"All right, if you're sure it's all right with Patty."

Alicia hugged him and covered him snugly with the warm quilt.

"She'll be really pleased. She'd die laughing if she came home and saw that old ghost of a tree waiting for her."

"Mo-om," Eddie protested, trying to keep a straight face. Then they all laughed.

As she walked from his room, Alicia thought about Patty. She'll be all right, she told herself. But she didn't believe it.

11:05 P.M.

Roger heard the tart, persistent buzzing. He groped for the plastic box. Only when he closed his hand around it did he realize that the sound had come from the television set—not the hospital's paging system. He gasped for breath. His skin felt taut, stretched tightly over his flesh. Catching his breath, he got up and walked to the kitchen, feeling a gnawing hunger. He looked into the refrigerator. It was stocked with all the basics of a healthy diet—for normal people. Greens, red and yellow vegetables, fruits. All were things he couldn't eat: all the food that contained phosphorous and potassium, minerals his kidneys would not tolerate.

Why did Martha buy all this crap when she knew she wouldn't be home to eat it herself? She knew how little he could eat of healthy stuff. But of course, he realized, she had bought it because they had expected house guests last weekend. But their child's tonsillitis had forced Jason and Ruthy to cancel at the last moment. Roger had been relieved when they called. He wanted to see old friends, of course, but he didn't have the energy to play host for a whole weekend. Now all this stuff he couldn't eat gawked at him from the refrigerator.

In his frustration, he slammed the refrigerator door, but it sprang open again, jolting loose a bottle of salad dressing, which flew off a door shelf, ricocheted against the metal edge of a glass shelf, and splattered across the floor.

Roger fell to his knees, looked at the mess his anger had created, and doubled over with a long, guttural roar which turned to racking sobs. This was all too much. He'd had enough. This would never be over; kidney patients can be kept alive for years through dialysis—merely existing in this state of limbo. Was there any point in living if this was what life was to be like?

Then, as suddenly as the rage burst forth, it was gone. Enough with the self pity. He cleaned up the floor and the splatters on the refrigerator and adjacent cupboards. When all was spotless, he walked to the living room and straightened the evening papers. He took the stack of mail to his desk in the study, sorted bills from junk mail and threw his refuse in the waste basket. He neatly stacked Martha's collection of bulk mail at one corner of the desk. He wrote checks and prepared envelopes for mailing.

Then, with deliberate steps, he walked to the étagère on the far wall of the study. He reached his hand over the top trim and retrieved his dad's service revolver, the only memento he had from the old man's long career with the police department. He checked the chambers: loaded, as he remembered. He carried the gun back to the living room and sat down in his favorite chair next to the phone and answering machine—and the pager. He studied the gun, remembering how his dad used to clean and polish it every week.

"No, I never had to kill anyone, Roggie," his father once said. "I don't think I could." The old man had stroked the gun as he spoke.

"This gun has saved my life, and scared off men who wanted my blood. But guns should never be used to kill people."

Good thing you're not a cop today, Roger thought. He caressed the gun, wanting to feel his father's touch again. He set the gun on his lap and turned his attention to the programming compartment of the answering machine, mentally practicing his new message several times, perfecting the wording. Dryness clutched his throat, and he felt himself trembling. Butterflies, everyone called them. He regained control, cleared his throat and pushed the record button.

11:10 P.M.

The sound of the steady, piercing tone filled the room. Everyone stared at the monitors, especially the EEG. It was flat. Brain function appeared to have stopped permanently. After releasing a long breath, Hartung laid down the probe he had been holding, dropped his face mask, and removed his protective goggles.

"There's nothing left, he announced."

Becky draped a towel over Donald Mills's head. Hartung looked at the young intern who had asked to watch the surgery. The kid looked pretty green, but, after turning away for a couple of good breaths, he looked back to the table again. Now he also dropped his mask and removed the glasses, looking thankful for a free intake of air.

"Are you all right?" Hartung asked. "The first time this happens is always the hardest." He hoped the young fellow didn't think he was talking down to him.

"These get to be routine after a while, but they're never pleasant."

The younger man shook his head slowly. He looked at Hartung, then back to the drape.

"Why did you bother? Why all the urgency for a 'next of kin' to authorize surgery when—"

"When it was obvious there wasn't a damn thing we could do for the patient?" Hartung completed his thought. "And even if we could have saved him, he'd probably prefer to be dead, rather than survive brain damaged and with nothing left of his face?"

The intern looked surprised by the bluntness; his face flushed a deep red.

"That's the same question I asked years ago after watching my first one," Hartung said. The intern looked relieved.

"Granted Donald Mills was not likely to ever return to 'normal' again. The damage to his head was so pervasive. But we had to give him every chance. You'd be surprised at some of the ones we do bring back—though sometimes I'm not sure we're doing them a real favor. Still, some—especially a parent of a young family—will go through anything to have a few more years with their children. So that's not up to us to decide. This patient showed some heart and respiratory function when we got him in. So we put him on a ventilator and did everything we could to save his life.

"So, what happens now?" Smith asked.

"That's entirely up to the aunt. I hope she will decide to donate his organs. They appear to be very strong. First, however, the patient has to be declared dead—or brain dead. There are criteria for both."

Smitty and the residents seemed transfixed.

"Determination of cause of death is necessary for the certification of death. However, in accidents such as this one, where the damage is sustained almost exclusively to the head, there is potential for harvesting viable organs for transplant. But, first, before we approach the family for that, there has to be the determination of brain death."

Smitty nodded. "So, he's brain dead now?"

"Actually, no. Not in the legal sense."

"Meaning?"Burk asked.

"That we have to go through a process of assurance before we can declare Donald Mills legally brain dead. It will only take about a half hour. Are any of you up for that?"

Three faces told the answer louder than their voices.

"Let's take ten minutes, people," the surgeon said, "then we'll reconvene to finish the job." All but Becky left the OR hurriedly. She would monitor the patient through the testing and until the procurement coordinator arrived.

Step by step, Hartung moved through the required tests, checking for the possibility of reversible brain stem damage, like the presence of intoxicants—heavy amounts of drugs or alcohol—or hypothermia, the body having been shut down due to prolonged exposure to cold temperatures. Next followed tests for brain stem reflexes. Next they proceeded on to check evidence of spontaneous respiration. Each procedure Hartung explained and carried out brought further amazement to his young observers.

"I had no idea all this was involved." Burk said.

"We have to cover all the bases to protect the right to life of this patient, and every other one who dies like him—before we seek permission for organ donation."

"Do you think he will become an organ donor?" asked Smitty.

"That's very hard to predict, in the absence of a donor card. Even with one, it depends upon the family. This can be a tough decision for the next of kin to face when they have just experienced such shocking loss. But, because it's so important, we'll ask."

Finally the patient had to be tested for ability to sustain unassisted breathing. All eyes had been focused on the patient, waiting for what seemed like an eternity for this final test of respiratory function. Attention darted from the patient to the timing clock. When the wait was finally over, Hartung checked his own watch, and in a barely audible voice, announced:

"Patient Donald Mills is brain dead. Time noted: eleven fifty P.M." Hartung turned to Becky. "Will you call LifeLine?"

"Will do," Becky answered, and left the room.

14

MIDNIGHT

12:00 A.M.

The persistent ringing of her phone dragged Carolyn Ames out of her dream. This better not be some drunk calling a wrong number, she thought, as she groped for the telephone.

"Hi, Carolyn. This is Becky down at Met. General. We have a potential organ donor—an accident victim. His name is Donald Mills."

Carolyn groped to turn on the light and, wide awake, sat up. The digital clock indicated 12:05. She calculated her usual allowance for the five minutes fast setting. She'd done this with her alarm clock since nursing school.

"Solid organs?"

"Practically new issue."

"Has anyone talked to the family yet?" She put on her watch as she held the phone with her shoulder.

"Tom Hartung is on his way out to break the news to the victim's family. The only next of kin is a ninety-year-old aunt.

"How do you know her age?"

"The reception clerk asked out of curiosity."

"I'll be there. Thanks for the call, Becky."

Carolyn invariably became wide awake when these calls came, even in the middle of the night. It had been two years since she'd hung up her nursing whites and took the job as a coordinator for LifeLine, the area regional procurement center, and she still felt excitement whenever the call clanged. Like a Dalmatian, she always said; once the alarm sounded, she was ready to go to the fire. Her clothes were hung over her chair, shoes and stockings alongside, a practice she had begun her first night on call.

Quickly she dressed, ran into the bathroom to clean up, applied a little lipstick and brushed her brown hair.

The phone calls usually came from several hospitals, though the major trauma centers were her primary sources. Their patients tended to be younger and more healthy at the time of death. When she had taken on this role, she'd settled into an apartment with freeway proximity to all of them. It was important to get to the families before they gave up in despair and went home. Within ten minutes, she was ready and locking her apartment door.

Carolyn ran down the stairs—the elevator was too slow—and out toward her car.

As she hurried, she noticed the unseasonably warm night and was thankful. Certainly it was better than trying to warm up a cold car. Putting her key in the ignition, she thought excitedly of the lives that might be saved. As she drove, she began to practice her presentation for Donald Mills's elderly aunt.

12:10 A.M.

A doctor was walking toward them. Lying on her side, Margaret couldn't tell if this was the one she'd talked to earlier.

She scrambled to sit up, with Michael's help. The doctor crouched in front of them.

"Mrs. Bond?" Yes, the voice was the same. She nodded.

The doctor looked at Margaret and then at Michael.

"Are you a member of the family?"

Before he could answer, Margaret spoke.

"He is my nephew's closest friend." Michael gently put his hand on Margaret's arm.

The doctor reached out to Michael. "I'm Dr. Hartung, Mr. Mills's attending physician." He turned back to Margaret.

"I'm afraid the news is very bad. The cranial damage was massive. We still have him on assisted breathing now, but he is brain-dead." Margaret had heard the term—newspaper, television, perhaps. But she had never paid much attention. One doesn't, she thought, if it doesn't affect you. What did it mean? It surely couldn't apply to Donald—not to her Donald. Panic was rising into her throat. She felt unable to take the next breath. Michael's grip tightened on her arm. She sensed it was hurting, but she actually felt nothing. She watched him staring at the doctor in disbelief. Tears seeped from his eyes.

"There must be something you can do. Please!" The panic in Michael's voice startled Margaret.

"I'm sorry. But we did everything we could for your friend. You must believe that."

Margaret laid her hand on Michael's hand—as much for his comfort as for her own.

"I'm very sorry to have to burden you further, Mrs. Bond, but we need a positive identification on Mr. Mills. Would you—?"

"I'll do it, doctor," Michael said.

They left together, and Margaret tried to understand. Don't they know if this is really Donald? She thought the library book and knowing he was missing was all they needed. But now they still had to know for sure. Oh God, please, couldn't it be some other man?" She prayed.

12:15 A.M.

"This is very difficult for Mrs. Bond, I'm sure," the doctor said to Michael as they moved down the softly lit corridor. "It's always hard to give such news to the family, but it's really hard for this poor woman."

Michael nodded. "She has no one else." He tried to tell himself he was up to doing whatever identification they needed, but the truth was he was not doing well at all. However, he couldn't allow Mrs. Bond to do this.

"By the way, I'm Tom Hartung."

"I'm Michael Fredericks. Donald was on his way to my house when this happened."

"I'm very sorry." The words sounded perfunctory, but Michael supposed an emergency room surgeon had to say them much too often. Yet his expression showed compassion.

Dr. Hartung stepped in front of Michael as they approached a surgical room, ablaze with light. He looked in and then steered Michael off to the side, away from the door.

"They're just about finished cleaning up in there. We can wait until they are done." He squatted next to Michael's wheelchair, a gesture Michael always appreciated.

"Have you been in this chair long?"

"Since I graduated high school. A bad dive into a swimming pool. I was lucky I didn't lose everything."

"Those things can happen in the blink of an eye." The doctor nodded, understanding. "Were you and Mr. Mills long time friends?"

"Since second grade. And that's a long time." He felt himself smiling for a moment—then remembered what lay ahead.

A man in a light green uniform passed through the door, pushing a cart loaded with a pair of large trash containers, a pail, mops, and an assortment of cleaning bottles. He reached back to the wall, and dimmed the lights.

"It's okay now, Dr. Hartung. Sorry it took so long."

"No problem, Charlie. And thanks."

The doctor led the way. Michael took a long, deep breath and let it out before following.

The room was stark white. The high voltage lights were off, but it was still bright. On an operating table the form of a body was visible under a large sheet. A nurse stood next to several pieces of equipment, apparently checking readings.

"How're we doing, Becky?" the doctor asked.

"He's still stabilized." She did not look back at either of them, but continued studying and regulating the digital lights and graphs.

"Good. Did you reach Carolyn yet?"

"She's on her way." The nurse turned and left the room.

Dr. Hartung looked at Michael. "His face was badly injured. What about his hair?"

Michael closed his eyes to rub out the picture of the covered body. "Brown, light brown. Almost blond. Slightly receding on each side."

The doctor moved to the head of the table and folded the sheet back slightly, away from the edge of the patient's hairline. "Does this look right?"

Michael reluctantly moved himself alongside. The top of the head was also wrapped. "I guess so. It's all wet and slicked back, so it's hard to be sure. But I think it's him."

"Any marks or unusual characteristics elsewhere on his body that you can remember?"

Michael thought. Then he remembered the scar above Donald's knee.

"His left leg, just above the knee. Donny cut himself once. He'd gotten a pocket knife from his Uncle Paul. Donny was showing off and jabbed the thing right into his leg. It took several stitches to close it. I laughed every spring when I saw him in shorts for the first time. That scar was still there."

For just an instant Michael held onto hope that there would be no scar, that it wasn't Donald after all. Then the doctor walked around the other side of the table to the left side and lifted the sheet just enough for the silver-white scar to appear.

"Like this?"

"Yes, sir. That's it." He nodded. It was Donald. He could not hold back the tears.

Margaret looked at the doctor, not comprehending where his words were going. Her mind tried to work. She saw Michael, now with locked focus on the doctor, nodding his response. So she, too, nodded, without comprehension.

"Mrs. Bond. I know this is a difficult time for you, but, though your nephew is dead, others' lives might be saved. All of your nephew's injuries are to the head, which means he is a very good candidate to be an organ donor. We've called one of the people involved in this program to come and visit with you—if that's all right with you."

Michael's eyes were squeezed shut, and tears trickled down his cheeks. But he was nodding. Margaret wanted the relentless pain to be over. Now it was becoming worse. Was Donald really dead? What had the doctor said about organs? Donald's organs? Michael and the doctor were looking at her. They expected an answer. But what was the question? She hadn't heard the question.

Michael turned his face squarely toward her. "Donald is dead, Mrs. Bond. His body is being kept alive by machines that make him breathe to help his heart continue beating." He glanced at the doctor for agreement. "Soon they will have to turn off the machines. But they can operate on him before that time, and his heart, his kidneys, whatever else, can be removed from his body and given to someone else who is seriously ill, to people who will die without that new heart or liver." Again he glanced briefly at the doctor and back to Margaret.

"But, Michael, we can't let them cut up Donald and give parts of him away."

Michael looked to the doctor again—this time pleading for help.

"Mrs. Bond. Right now, I'm not asking for you to agree to this surgery. I'm just asking you to talk with a young woman who works with the donor program and can explain it better for you. She will tell you about the process and the need for these organs. Then you are free to say no if you do not want this for your nephew."

Margaret looked at Michael. "Should we do this?"

"Who'll get the organs?" Michael asked.

"We don't know yet," the doctor said.

"All they want you to do, Mrs. Bond, is talk with the woman. Then you can say yes or no. Doesn't that sound fair?"

Margaret nodded, then looked at the doctor and nodded again. She would talk to whomever they sent, but she was sure it would never be the right thing to do. Donald deserved to rest in peace. He shouldn't be operated on and have parts removed for *who knows what.*

The doctor stood up and returned the chair to its place. Then he crouched down in front of her.

"I'm so terribly sorry, Mrs. Bond," he said. "I know you loved your nephew very much, and you will suffer his loss for a long time. Whatever you decide, I can promise we will treat his body with the utmost respect."

After shaking hands with Michael, he walked away.

Margaret stared after him, imagining she saw him still walking long after he had been erased by the large swinging doors.

Something was terribly wrong here. She wanted to ask Michael, but he, too, was watching those same doors. His face was crumbling. But what could she do? What was she supposed to do?

Her eyes were open, but no longer saw. Panic churned her stomach. Then she became aware that Michael was looking at her.

"Mrs. Bond, how would you feel about my calling Father John? He's a good friend of yours, isn't he?"

"Yes, but I don't want to bother him at this time of night. Gracious, it's past midnight, isn't it?"

"But, he's your friend—and mine. We need him." The words of anguish startled her. Sometimes she had almost forgotten Michael was here, let alone that he was suffering this atrocity as well as she was.

"He would want to be here."

"If you're sure."

Michael nodded and went to make the call

12:25 A.M.

As Alicia washed her face before going to bed, she noticed a smile on the reflection in the mirror. The laughter with David and Eddie had felt good. It was the first time since Christmas she'd smiled. Even over the holidays, when Patty was home, it was not the same as past Christmases. The happiness was forced; she really wanted to cry.

Tonight the laughter had been a wonderful tonic for all three of them, and certainly for her mother, too. The smile in the mirror gave her hope that she could hang on to some thread of reality. A strand of faith.

"Thank you, God, for helping us get through this."

When she got into bed, David was still awake. She was indeed blessed to have this wonderful person so faithfully beside her, sharing the load. He didn't talk a lot, but, when he did speak, he was well worth listening to. Her smile again came naturally.

"You really pulled off the Christmas tree caper beautifully," she said. "I didn't know what I was going to do."

He reached for her. "How long has it been since I told you I love you, Alie?"

"Much, much too long," she said.

The warmth of his body wrapping her in love brought her to tears. Not tears of sorrow, but a joyous frenzy that blocked all thought of these past weeks' barren nights. She was alive again.

"Oh, Alie, don't cry." His voice was soft and breathless. "This is good and right."

"I know, sweet David." She locked her legs around him, holding him, wanting never to let go.

15

A PLEA FOR LIFE

12:30 A.M.

Michael hung up the receiver and his tense shoulders felt normal again. Father John would be here shortly. It wasn't that Michael was a coward about facing death, in fact, many times he had become weary of life after all these years of dealing with his useless legs. But he was a stranger to Mrs. Bond and certainly not the one to tell her what she should do at a time like this. He hoped the priest would get here before the transplant woman arrived.

He maneuvered his wheel chair back in Mrs. Bond's direction, but stopped short of going to her side. She seemed to have dozed off. Poor woman. This must be a stunning shock for her—as it was for him.

He could not remember what she looked like when he and Donny were children. Nor did she look like the woman he had pictured when Donald spoke of her. She was so small, a small and wrinkled form, still bundled up in her winter coat. Her eyes held a kind and gentle look. That did surprise him. Donny could be mean-spirited in the way he talked about people, including his aunt. His off-handed comments about Mrs. Bond certainly created a different picture than he was seeing now. The guy was so protective of his privacy that he never wanted Michael to see his aunt Margaret—though he had once. It seemed so long ago. At Donny's mother's funeral, Donny had pushed his wheelchair away so quickly that Michael had hardly seen her. Donny always sounded as if he suspected she was some sort of a spy, trying to discover secret truths about him. Michael had known this paranoia was ridiculous. But he never said anything. He couldn't jeopardize their friendship. Besides, he never knew for sure when Donny was telling the real truth about anything unscientific. To Donald, science was the only objective certainty. All else was a matter of subjective reality.

However, though Donny would never admit it, Michael was certain his friend had loved his aunt. When she was out of town, he really missed her. Maybe what he really missed were those home-cooked dinners he always talked about her making every night. She even cooked meals for him to warm when she wasn't going to be home for a night or so. Donald complained that she fussed over him too much, but she had once been hospitalized and Donald had been nearly frantic with worry. That's when Michael realized that this woman was more a mother to Donny than a bothersome aunt. When his real mother died, Donny had taken it very hard—though no one at the services would have guessed. He wore a mask of stoicism that never broke until late the night of the funeral. Michael had been sleeping when Donald came pounding at his door. It was the only time Michael ever saw his friend drunk. And only that once, after too much booze, did Donald allow the tears to break loose. He had slept it off on Michael's couch, and, in the morning, he bristled when Michael had hinted at what happened the night before. But, from that time, Michael always recognized when his friend was hurting. Sarcasm and ridicule might slide across every word, yet

Michael knew. He always heard the undercurrent of sadness, disappointment, or fear.

When Donald had returned from New York, Mrs. Bond welcomed him home. Michael had envied Donny that. His own family had been a broken home. Following a divorce, his father had taken Michael's older brother and they had both disappeared. His mother was overwhelmed by her loss. She couldn't deal with her own anguish, let alone recognize Michael's. He was only eight at the time, but he quickly realized he had to become the man of the house if either of them was to survive.

Only after Michael's accident, the summer he graduated from high school, did his mother muster the energy to face reality. She was a real mother for nearly four years, pushing him to do his physical therapy, getting him to his college classes. Then it was time for him to become the parent again as he watched her long, painful death from liver cirrhosis. After that, he had no one to care about him. Even worse, he himself had no one to care about. It would have been nice, he thought, to have someone like this good, gentle woman be concerned if he were alive or dead. But the agony of loving someone comes when that someone is lost. Michael knew all about that.

12:35 A.M.

Dr. Tom Hartung looked at his watch as Carolyn Ames ran into the staff lounge across from the surgical suites.

"What took you so long?"

He always said that. She knew it had been exactly thirty-one minutes since she'd hung up the phone.

"Sorry. My car needed a tune-up." Becky looked from Carolyn to her boss and hooted. Carolyn knew she could expect Hartung's wry questions whenever he was on rotation when she rolled in late at night. She usually spent the driving time to prepare some new response for him. It relaxed her mind for the stress that lay ahead. She slowed her movements for a mere second to watch for his smile and was rewarded.

Then, she quickly hung up her coat and stepped into a scrub suit, a plain, green, two-piece suit that was standard now for nearly everyone staffing the emergency room.

"What have we got?" she asked, pulling on a lab coat to cover the blue turtleneck sweater she had worn under the uniform shirt. This place was always so cold.

Hartung handed her the chart.

"Male, fortyish" he said. She followed him into the OR as he talked. "Riding a bicycle when he was hit head-on by a small van."

Carolyn shuddered as he just barely lifted the white sheeting draped over the patient's head. "They say he was something of a recluse. Lived in an apartment above his aunt."

"The ninety-year-old?"

"Yeah, that's the tough part. She was very close to him, and she's understandably bewildered."

"And the major organs?"

"No apparent trauma from impact or the fall. His aunt indicated on the intake form that he rarely smoked or drank. She told the desk attendant he didn't drive a car, rode his bike or walked everywhere. Excellent muscle tone. I'd say he's in great shape."

"Previous medical history?"

"We've got a gap there. His history looks fine, but she said she wasn't sure on some aspects. Mother died of cancer, but the father died from heart attack years ago. About fifty at the time. However, his heartbeat has remained solid throughout."

Carolyn scanned the chart's notations. He certainly looked good as a donor. "All labs so far are normal?" she asked.

"Clean as a whistle."

"All right!" Carolyn felt a rush of excitement. There were long waiting lists—men, women and children—who needed each of these organs. She pulled up the computer files listing top candidates for each organ—all so much in need. Tonight she could reconnect life to four lucky people.

She added a consent form to the chart, then turned abruptly toward the Emergency waiting room, waving over her shoulder.

"Wish me luck."

Before pushing through the double doors, she stopped to review the paper work she carried. She always wanted to know everything about the patient, firsthand, before facing the family. It helped the family make that tough decision if they saw that she cared about their lost member.

12:45 A.M.

Michael had steadily watched the entrance to the Emergency Room. He should have been trying to help Mrs. Bond, but instead he seemed to be hanging on by a mere thread, drowning in his own pain. He wished for some easy way to pull loose from the thread, to go where Donny had gone.

Finally a familiar figure came rushing through the Emergency Room door.

"Father John. Thank god," murmured Michael.

Margaret awakened with a jolt, and was blanketed in the embrace of the young priest and dear friend.

"Oh, Margaret, I am so sorry."

Father John turned to hug Michael. No words were needed. Michael realized that there was, after all, someone for him to hang on to.

The priest ran his hand through his ruffled, black hair and sat next to Margaret.

"He can't be dead," she said, imploring one of them to verify her hope. "This can't be. I was the one who was supposed to die first. I'm an old woman; I'm ready to go, not Donald." She seemed to be talking to herself, but she drew a deep breath and continued.

"And now," she said, slowly shaking her head, "They want to do an operation, and take his parts—his organs—and give them away to somebody else. That's not right, is it, Father? He should be buried as he is, shouldn't he?"

The priest looked directly at her. "That's not a simple question, Margaret. Do you remember in the Bible when Jesus said there was no greater love than when someone gave his life for another?" She nodded. "Well, Donald is dead. There is nothing that can bring him back to us. This seems such a senseless death, but maybe it can have some reason, after all. If Donald's organs can give others life, isn't that what the Bible teaches?"

"Oh, I don't know. I am so tired and so confused. Is this really the right thing to do? Are you sure?"

"Yes, Margaret, it is right. Other people may die, needlessly, if we don't do this for them. Leaders of all major religious groups, including the Pope, have spoken out that donating organs is a good and proper thing to do."

Margaret sat quietly, eyes down, unable to comprehend these answers. Each man held a hand. "I don't want him mutilated, all cut up."

"Margaret, the Donald you knew is no longer in that body. The part of him that you love has already gone to heaven."

She looked at him, both puzzled and relieved. "Do you think that can be? Do you think he can really be in heaven—after so long away from God?"

"He was never away from God, Margaret." Father John smiled at her. "He just thought he was. God doesn't let go that easily."

"Mrs. Bond," Michael said, "I wanted to wait until you had time to think this through, but Donald wanted his organs to be used this way. We had talked about it." Margaret studied him with surprise. "He thought it was morally wrong to let organs go to the grave when others needed them to live. That's exactly how he said it."

Margaret closed her eyes. Both men waited.

She opened her eyes slowly, staring directly ahead of her. When her voice came, it was soft, but clear.

"Then I guess that is how it should be."

16

THE LONG NIGHT CONTINUES

1:00 A.M.

From a distance, Carolyn thought the woman looked much younger than ninety years old. She was sitting with two younger men, one in a wheel chair. Age indeterminate. He appeared to be in shock. The second was younger, rumpled clothing and black hair. The other two were obviously leaning upon him emotionally. They all looked up as she approached. She leaned down to speak.

"Mrs. Bond? I'm Carolyn White. I work with LifeLine, the organ procurement agency." Slow down, she told herself. Keep it simple. She looked at the men seated beside the aunt. They were studying her. She felt saddened for all three of them. She turned to the man in the wheelchair.

"Are you also a relatives of Mr. Mills's?" she asked.

"No. I'm Michael. Donald is my friend. He was on his way to my house." His voice cracked and she saw the hard-held tears.

"And I'm Father John Jackson, a friend of the family." She shook the priest's hand, then brought a chair into their circle.

She focused on the aunt, but kept the friends in sight. "I am so sorry for your loss, Mrs. Bond. I hope you can believe that Dr. Hartung did everything he could to save Donald's life."

All three nodded.

"I believe Dr. Hartung told you that I would be coming to talk to you about the organ donor program. Have you previously heard anything about organ donation?"

Again Margaret nodded—a slow, almost rhythmic nod. "Yes, I've heard something about it before tonight—only a little, actually. But Father John and Michael have been explaining it to me."

"Then you probably know it is possible to take good strong organs from someone who has died—usually accident or gun-shot victims who have no further chance to live—and transplant them into terminally ill patients, giving them another chance at life."

She paused to read their reactions. Not much to read with Mrs. Bond yet. Poor old woman, must be stunned with grief. But the men were nodding; at least they understood. Margaret, however, looked confused.

"Is there anything you'd like to ask me, Mrs. Bond?" Carolyn said sympathetically.

"I don't understand. The doctor said Donald was some kind of dead. Or is he really still alive?"

"When Donald was brought into the hospital, he was immediately put on a ventilator, a respirator that acts as a breathing machine. And he began to receive medications and fluids to keep him alive while Dr. Hartung operated on him to try to save his life. All of this kept his heart beating and his organs functioning."

The woman was nodding. So far, so good. "Because all of Donald's injuries were to his head, tests were used to measure the activity in his brain, the brain waves, as they are called." Again Mrs. Bond nodded.

"During the operation, Dr. Hartung tried to repair the damage to Donald's head, but it was impossible to do enough. The brain wave monitor and further tests have indicated there is no sign of any activity in your nephew's brain. The brain is dead. Medically and legally, Donald is dead.

"However, the ventilator has been left running, and so Donald's body acts as if it were alive and working on its own. Nevertheless, he is brain dead. Once we turn off the machines— and we will have to turn them off in time—Donald's body will be dead, also.

"Does this help you to understand, Mrs. Bond?"

The woman nodded slowly. But a question remained in the slight lowering of her eyebrows.

"Who would get the organs if I give the permission?"

"Mrs. Bond, there are many people who are close to death tonight because their diseased organs—heart, kidneys, liver— are failing. If you allow us to give Mr. Mills's healthy organs to them, those patients can recover and go back to a full life with their families." Carolyn had no idea if she was reaching this poor, frightened woman.

"We are deeply sorry that nothing could be done to save your nephew, but at least you would know that his heart will live on in someone else's body. The same can be true for his liver, and his two kidneys. Four people's lives can be saved tonight with your nephew's organs."

The priest placed his hand on Mrs. Bond's arm and she nodded.

"Where do I sign? she asked. She signed the consent form for the four major organs. Carolyn wished she could get assign-ment for other tissue, also—bones and cartilage for damaged joints, skin transplants for burn victims. But she would not press this poor woman who was already so dazed with shock and loss. She was well satisfied to have a signature for the four strong, major organs.

"I know I can speak for the four fortunate people who will start new lives tonight, since we keep their names and locations confidential. For them and their families, thank you so very much for your kindness and generosity."

Carolyn turned to leave, but she had almost forgotten. "Mrs. Bond, we'll have your nephew's body moved to a quiet room in a short while. The young woman at the desk will let you know. Then you may want to spend some time in visitation." She would have stopped, but thought perhaps an explaination was in order. "Please, let me caution you, Donald's body will look quite normal. Of course, we will have his injuries draped, but his chest will rise and fall, as if breathing. His body will have good color and feel warm. But that is because of the ventilator and the medications still being administered.

"Again, let me thank you." Then she turned away.

That was always the hardest part. The families wanted to see their loved one fully clothed and looking as if he were resting peacefully. But head-injury fatalities rarely allowed open caskets. If the family wanted to spend a few minutes in quiet grieving, they would carry that grim picture always in their hearts. But at least donor families and friends knew that something of this person they loved would live on.

As she passed the ER admitting desk clutching the clip board and signed papers, Carolyn sighed deeply, finally allowing a feeling of satisfaction to spread through her. Her work, however, was just beginning.

Tom Hartung, the attending physician up to this point, signed off on the patient. Donald Mills, kept alive only by ventilator and IVs, was now, in effect, Carolyn's patient. She first wrote the standing orders for the organ donor cadaver. There were specific protocols for each organ, and they had to work in harmony to keep all organs vital until time for transplant. She ordered the specific blood work needed for matching.

However, there were some uncertainties in Donald Mills's

medical history. This could be problematic. Carolyn wanted to talk with her medical director—just to be safe. She hated ruining Emily's sleep, but if four people were going to go through the trauma of transplant surgeries, Emily would want to be very sure they received strong, healthy organs.

Carolyn dialed the pager number, then waited for the call-back.

1:30 A.M.

Emily McCabe felt the pulsing of her pager through the pillow. That meant only one thing: LifeLine had an available donor. While being awakened in the middle of the night was never a picnic, she came to life quickly, and was thankful for the soundless call of her new pager. She'd hated the shrillness of a phone shrieking in the middle of the night. Every time it rang, her husband Glen woke up and reminded her that now he would-n't get back to sleep again "after all that commotion." Sometimes the kids had been roused, too—scared to pieces. One of us awake around here in the middle of the night is quite enough, Emily thought. As she pulled on her robe and slippers and walked to her study to return the page, she felt that surge of elation that always came with the prospect of another organ donor. Some very lucky patients would be infused with new life tonight.

"Yes, Carolyn, what do you have?"

"A middle-aged unmarried male. Riding a bicycle; hit head-on by a van. Tom Hartung worked on him, but there was lit-tle chance with the extent of brain injury."

Emily sighed. These cases had never toughened her.

"Heck of a way to go," she responded.

"It sure is. But, fortunately for donor purposes, the injuries to the rest of the body appear minor. He looks to be in excellent shape, so Hartung signed off. I've started all the routine drips. However, there are some gaps in his medical history, and his father died of a heart attack in his fifties. No signs thus far in the patient. He was extremely fit physically, and his heart is maintaining beautifully. The next of kin, who worked on the medical history and gave permission, is an elderly aunt. Really hurting."

"Anything available from his regular physician?"

"He had no physician. He didn't believe in doctors."

"Smart man." They both laughed. "All right, run the standard ECG and serology work. Pay particular attention to HIV and drug tests. Keep an eye on the monitors, and call me back when you have the results."

"Will do. You can go back to sleep now." Emily heard the chuckle at the other end of the line.

"Sure I can." Another audible laugh.

Emily curled up on the couch in her study, wishing she could fall back to sleep. But her battery was charged now. She traded the couch for her recliner and pulled the crossword puzzle out of yesterday's paper. At least that might stabilize her equilibrium. Initially the lure for this position as medical director for the organ procurement center was that it had been part time, providing more opportunity to be home with Glen and the kids. They were the priority right now. But the drama of this work quickly got into Emily's blood. And the turbulent—behind the scenes—races with time vitalized her.

Unfortunately, the havoc of drunken driving, guns, and gang fights was not something that could be boxed into part-time hours. Over the holidays the flood of potential donors from party goers made the job nearly full time work, and on the night shift at that. However, after the beginning of the new year, as usual, the job had slowed down again as the world succumbed to bill-paying and staying warm. Everyone at LifeLine breathed easier, and caught up on sleep and comp days. Also, her coordinators had become so competent at their jobs that her tasks were much more advisory than hands on. But there were still occasions, as she suspected tonight might be, when she was needed at the

hospital for a medical judgement which her staff was not authorized to make.

At least Emily was thankful she didn't have to rotate in the
emergency room—as Tom Hartung had chosen to do—dealing
with trauma care of these victims. Her role came into play after
heroic surgery had failed, and after donor permissions had been
granted. As medical director her job was different from any medicine she'd ever done during her nearly fifteen years of school
and practice.

Emily remembered her tenure in cardiology. Often then
she had been on the waiting end—hoping for an available organ
for a patient she could no longer save with conventional medicine. But after her second baby, she realized that for her the rig-
ors of a full time practice would conflict with the mothering her
children needed for the next few years. Then she happened upon
this opening and was hooked.

Actually she had been hooked once before, but made the
tough decision to get unhooked. She'd been doing her final
cardiology residency back when the second round of heart
transplants began in the early eighties. The miracle discovery of
immunosuppressant drugs, like Cyclosporine, meant that recipients no longer automatically rejected their new organs. It was
the dawn of a new era in medicine, and Emily had seriously
considered going on into cardiac surgery. But after much soul-
searching, she decided she'd been studying to be a doctor long
enough. It was time to be a doctor. So she joined a diagnostic
group as the new, young, and female cardiology whiz. However,
the fascination of transplantation never left her. So, when this
job opened up, the decision was easy enough to make. Again
tonight she was sure it was the right one.

17

A HEART FOR RUDY

The donor's preliminary reports came back clean. Everything looked good. No HIV nor indication of drug use—not even alcohol. The latest ECG looked normal. Carolyn phoned the encouraging reports to McCabe, who was equally satisfied.

"However, we do have one small problem," Carolyn explained. "Medical Examiner Balland is rattling around. The vehicle that struck our man was a truck owned by some big corporation and Balland always seems to have his ear to the track. I've noticed before, with other potentially 'wrongful death' cases, that he seems to enjoy moonlighting as a professional witness. Tom Hartung doesn't want to antagonize him. This is Hartung's turf, but he's likely to have to work with Balland for the next trauma death and the next after that."

"No problem," Emily said. "I'll be glad to handle it. Besides, with that unknown family heart background, I probably should come in, if only to cover you. Crank up the organ listings and start your matching. Threaten everyone in-house with whatever it takes. If there are any further problems, I'll be there in about forty minutes. But we can't risk a good donor becoming unstable. If push gets to shove, don't wait for me."

"Will do."

Again Carolyn phoned the lab. A couple of standard reports were still missing. She poured a cup of coffee, burning her tongue on the first sip. Okay, C.A., she addressed herself, time to begin phase two.

Word that Emily was coming had quickly doused two fires. Carolyn informed Balland that *Doctor* Emily McCabe would soon be here to handle his concerns. He grudgingly accepted Tom Hartung's cause of death. Then Kurt Polanski, another surgeon, raised a flap searching for an operating room for an emergency appendectomy. He claimed this OR was his customary turf and had been tied up far too long with a brain-dead patient. Carolyn bit her tongue and reminded herself that Polanski was merely concerned about the immediate needs of his own patient. She hoped some physician would do the same for her if she had an emergency some day.

She again dropped the name—*Doctor* McCabe—who would be here shortly to resolve all such matters. In addition, Carolyn suggested that Polanski check on one of the hospital's outpatient surgical suites, since she was anticipating multiple harvesting and transplants tonight. He agreed and left. After that, she called scheduling to put a hold on all ORs in this wing.

"It may take as many as five, with heavy traffic between them," she said.

For now everyone waited quietly. At least the surgical staff did. Carolyn, however, paced the floor, anxious to get on with the night's work. "Why do lab results take so long when they are so critical to what needs to be done?" She murmured. A rhetorical take-off on the "watched pot" theory, she supposed.

She went to the computer, keying in information already

charted before and during the donor's surgery tonight: blood type, age, size, and weight data, cause of death. Finally, the remaining results came in, and Carolyn had enough for preliminary matching. She tore off the print-outs that gave her a listing of leading contenders—patients who matched the donor and who desperately needed these particular organs. This was the hard part. Every patient on any organ list was in critical need of a transplant.

As she surveyed the list, Carolyn saw two Status-One possibilities. One was in house; another was one hundred and sixty miles away, needing to come in to Metro Gen for his transplant.

Rudy Popovich, the latter, was the most at risk, not only because he was in end-stage heart failure, but also because his insurance problems had only been resolved for fifteen days. His time was quickly running out. There was a problem: the donor was considerably smaller than Mr. Popovich. It was time to telephone Dr. Jonah Dolan, ranked as the first person to be called. She gave him the good news.

"Both patients have good matching antigens. One, Mr. Nichols, is here; the other is Mr. Popovich in Duluth. The donor and Nichols are reasonably close in size and normal weight. Popovich, however, is over size recommendations. The donor weighs in at about one-forty, and the Duluth man's normal weight is about one-eighty-five." She paused to separate the issues. "To further complicate things, Macrae just reminded me yesterday that Mr. Popovich's insurance deadline is fast approaching. He now has about twenty-four hours of assured coverage on that HMO."

"I'd forgotten about that insurance problem." Dolan mused. "Poor guy must be frantic."

"His condition has been too critical to be frantic about anything but the present. But Macrae talks to his wife regularly, and the poor woman is major-league frantic."

"Refresh me. Has Mr. Popovich ever had any heart or chest surgery?"

"No surgeries. Not even a tonsillectomy."

"Well, I guess we could try for a heterotopic implant. That would allow us to use an undersized heart."

"Leaving his own heart in place, and attaching the donor organ to give it a kicker?"

"Yup. It's trickier than orthotopic—take one out and put one in. But this heart is too darned small for a man of Mr. Popovich's size. On the other hand, the hetero should give him the total pump capacity he needs for some years to come."

Carolyn waited for his thinking process to work through.

Dolan continued. "I think Nichols can hold on for a while yet. Worst case scenario, he can be on a balloon pump or a ventricular device for a few weeks until the next available donor comes along. However, those gadgets won't do a thing for Mr. Popovich if his insurance runs out before another heart is available. I think we have to try to give this one to him. Go ahead and notify Duluth. Then page Macrae. She's on for tonight, but she probably won't have the Duluth data at home, and we need to get started on that end.

The elation Carolyn felt at giving someone a new chance for life took hold of her. As she hung up the phone, she clenched a fist and raised it victoriously,

"Yes!" She shouted. A few minutes later, she was back on the telephone.

"Dr. Anderson, this is Carolyn Ames. I'm a transplant coordinator for LifeLine, calling from Metropolitan General. I'm sorry to wake you at this time of night, but we think we have a heart for your patient, Rudy Popovich."

The line seemed to go dead. Carolyn waited several seconds.

"It's a good match." This was no time for lengthy explanations about size. "With his insurance deadline, we consider him the best candidate."

The silence continued.

"Dr. Anderson, are you still there?"

"Yes, I'm sorry. I'm just trying to think. We're having a helluva blizzard up here. I got home at eleven from an emergency call at the hospital, and I could barely find my driveway."

"Wow. It's been fairly nice here today." She drew herself to attention. "We have another potential recipient who is also a good match. But Dr. Dolan particularly wants to give this one to Mr. Popovich, since this may be his last chance."

"Yes, his time is rather quickly winding down. There could be a court fight, but no assurances—even while the case goes to a judge."

"What's Mr. Popovich's condition right now?"

"He came into St. Louis County Hospital again a couple of weeks ago. I thought we'd lose him that night. But he pulled through once again. He's a tough guy, a lot of fight. I saw him about six tonight. He's stable, no fever or sign of infections. But his heart is very weak. I've got him on a monitor, of course, and a ventilator a good part of the time—and on isotropic drip, trying to keep him going so he could be ready at any time if there's a chance for a transplant. But he needs a new heart. We're losing him."

Carolyn listened and hoped.

"Let me make a few calls. There has to be some way to get him there. How much time do I have?"

Carolyn made a quick calculation. "We should have him here at the hospital in four hours. I'm sorry. I know this is difficult. I'll wait for your call."

Anderson's voice strengthened.

"Somehow we'll have him there. Count on it."

Next Carolyn dialed the paging number for a heart coordinator. Thank goodness Macrae was on tonight. The long trip would be iffy at best. She was glad Macrae always kept her cool in tough situations.

As soon as she had completed preparations for the heart transplant's arrival, Carolyn was back at the computer, drawing up the list of potential liver recipients.

18

THE ROLE OF CHANCE

1:45 A.M.

Emily McCabe had set the crossword puzzle aside. Not one word was completed. She'd pulled off two pieces of paper from the memo pad atop her desk—one for Glen, the other for Martha, the children's baby-sitter. The messages were similar, routine, nonspecific. She had learned some years back not to give precise times for her return. When she failed to meet the objective, it often created disappointment and sometimes anger. It was much safer to phone in updated reports. Dressing quickly and quietly, she left.

Now, as the garage door closed, she clicked on the car radio and slipped her favorite CD into the player. As she drove, she wondered where the recipients of tonight's donor organs were right now. How had they and their loved ones coped with the long days and nights of anxious waiting? Had they already made peace with what seemed to be the inevitable, or did they still passionately cling to hope? And what right did Carolyn and she have to play God and tell some patients "Yes," but turn their collective backs on the others, all the thousands of others.

Emily remembered the early days of transplant surgery,
when the failure rate was enormous for anyone but identical
twins. Kidneys were the only live donor organs that worked even
marginally. Everyone was certain that it was just a matter of time
before the rejection problem could be licked. But, until then,
transplantation came to a virtual halt.

So while we waited, she recalled, there was time to consider—on paper, at least—criteria for future decisions on which
patients would receive which organs. Emily was at a university in
New York at that time, and the chief resident gathered all the
cardiology residents together one day for what he called a "mercy
hearing." How, he asked them, can we ensure that the best candidate always got the organ? What standards would guarantee
fairness? Uncompromising dedication to absolute fairness was
the hallmark of that exercise. Total, unprejudiced equity must
be the only measure by which an organ recipient would be selected, they pronounced.

Emily slowed her small red BMW for the final turn leading out of the subdivision. Streets were quiet here late at night,
but traffic would increase as she headed toward the freeway and
down town. It was a different world she drove through in this
enclave, and a far different life from those earlier, struggling
years.

We were idealistic then, she remembered. It was all theory.
But, before long, other doctors would face the real decisions of
the real world of very ill patients who needed transplanted organs.

When Cyclosporine was finally available, real surgeons
had indeed struggled with those same issues and with the potential for corruption in the selection of the "most deserving."
Luckily the federal government got into the act back in 1984 and
set national standards. Of course, everyone hoped that the one
piece of legislation would solve the problems of organ allocation.
But it didn't. It still hadn't when Emily came aboard at LifeLine

last year. She found a myriad of national and local changes had been made over the intervening years since organ donation had been cranked up again. And each alteration, although created to safeguard the process, had made it more cumbersome. Emily remembered when only Status-One patients were eligible for a kidney transplant. And only patients who were in an ICU on a drip qualified as Status-One. Others might have been living with their lives on hold for years, waiting for a match. But, if they happened to be well enough to be home for a few days when a perfect organ became available, they lost their chance.

Emily talked to every surgeon in the region and drew up amended guidelines, which she had no trouble getting approved by participating doctors and hospitals. Now, patients are ranked on the list by how sick they are, how long they have been waiting, plus any critical, extenuating circumstances—such as Mr. Popovich's insurance problems.

Although the system wasn't perfect, with these hybrid factors they were usually able to make the best determinations on a per-case basis. Even her coordinators, and the surgeons and their transplant coordinators no longer complained about unfairness.

As she drew near to Met Gen, she turned off the stereo and scanned the area. She was entering the danger zone where an ambulance might be coming from any direction.

Henry, the night security guard, doffed his hat affably when she entered the parking lot.

"Evening, Dr. McCabe. I see you got the whole gang rounded up tonight."

She smiled and nodded. He's right about that. The gang's all here.

1:50 A.M.

Rudy Popovich's physician, Bob Anderson, was endeavoring to carry out his promise to Carolyn Ames that Rudy would be at the hospital when the donor heart arrived. Unfortunately, the raging blizzard was not complying.

"Hello, George. This is Bob Anderson. Sorry to call this time of night."

"No problem, Doc, what's happening?"

"Do you have any information on when this storm might let up? I've got a patient, Rudy Popovich, who needs to be in Minneapolis four hours from now—for a heart transplant."

"Oh, yeah. He's the one they did the story on in the papers." George made some clucking sounds. "I'm sorry, Doc, I checked with the weather guys less than an half hour ago. I've got a chopper stuck over in Bismarck. They don't expect any let up there until at least noon tomorrow."

"Damn. His time on that insurance business runs out in one more day. He has to get this heart or he's probably not going to make it."

"Better call Jerry Keenan with the State Highway Patrol, Doc. There's a chance he might be able to help you. I know he'll give it his best shot. Call him at home. Wait a minute." He left the phone, then came back and gave the doctor the number. "I'll keep in touch with the weather people, just in case there's any change. Good luck, Doc."

Anderson sighed deeply. We'll need it, he thought.

2:00 A.M.

It had been a rough day for Macrae Gorman, and it seemed it would never end. Potential heart recipients who were not presently confined to the hospital while waiting, along with in-house patients who were at least mobile, came in to the heart clinic for monitoring.

Many patients had come to know one another over their months of waiting. As they entered the waiting room, looking for familiar faces, each inquired about those missing. News of another transplant produced mixed feelings. Happiness for the recipient, but also touches of envy, often accompanied by guilt. But, generally, they kept hope alive for one another.

After the last appointment, Macrae had gone up to the cardiac wing to visit patients too ill to attend the clinic. Being a cheerleader was exhausting, she thought when she returned to the coordinator's office to work on her record-keeping. The day after tomorrow, Macrae would be leaving for a seminar in San Diego and a few days vacation. She wanted everything to be up to date. Her cohort, Beth, the other heart coordinator, would have double duty while Macrae was gone. The least she could do was to get everything in order for her. She worked on through dinner, which was a sandwich and soda from the vending machine.

After completing notations on ten in-patient files, she had come to the eleventh. Robert Macalester, age nineteen. First diagnosed in May of last year. Time on the list—five months. So terribly sad, Macrae thought. In June the principal of his high school and his homeroom teacher had presented him with his diploma in his ICU unit. A group of his classmates stood outside the ICU entrance and sang their school fight song. Robert's condition allowed him to leave the hospital three weeks later, returning again in August, when he'd been upgraded on the donor waiting list. From then on he bounced back every few weeks. At Christmas, he was well enough for a private room, and his parents and six brothers stayed the day in the waiting area, as one at a time spent quiet moments with Robert while he slept or when he was awake and alert enough to hear their teasing. The family seemed driven to believe his survival into this new year was a good omen. Surely now he'd get a new heart and live happily ever after. Such is the substance of dreams, but Robert was a mortal being.

He had died today, just an hour before Macrae made rounds on the floor. It had drained nearly every ounce of emotion she had to face that wounded family, able only to offer her sympathies. Life wasn't fair—to the Macalesters or the others who watched a loved one slip away before a heart could be found. This was the agony of Macrae's job.

As she made the final notations on the file, she felt very tired. She stamped Robert's file "Deceased" and dropped it on the secretary's desk as she headed toward the door. Almost as an after thought, she turned back, switched on the computer and called up the heart waiting list. Robert's name had been at the top for his blood group. So close, yet a lifetime away. Removing his name from the list seemed like wiping out his life. She wished it were as easy to wipe out the memories of that fine young man.

The next two named within blood type category were actually tied for position—one by the gravity of his condition, the other by severity, plus the quirk of an insurance problem. For a moment, she wished she weren't on call tonight, or else would be lucky and not have any calls. Then the choice would be faced while she was gone on her trip West.

Then she took back the wish.

Even though it was late, the dirty laundry had stared her in the face when she arrived home and went into the bathroom. She was too keyed up to sleep anyway. The laundry room was dark and dreary as she snapped on the light.

As always, she still wore her pager. Don't leave home without it was the first lesson she had learned when she moved over from cardiac floor nursing to join the multi-organ transplant team as a heart coordinator. These had been the four most wonderful, yet painful years of her career. The surgical teams were tops, as were all the coordinators and back-up people in both procurement and transplantation. They had chosen their positions because of a strong sense of mission, and there was a deep bond of kinship among everyone involved. She could never imagine leaving this team now—even with its heartbreaks.

She returned to her apartment with the last load of dry clothes. She still felt tired. Take ten, she told herself, then dumped both baskets on the bed to start folding.

That was when her beeper sounded.

"Swell," she muttered, and dialed the hospital on her bed-side phone. She knew what to expect, even before the call was answered. In all likelihood the race was on for two of her patients. Which one would win? This was supposed to be handled tomorrow night when she was no longer on call. But tomorrow was probably too late for Mr. Popovich. Who was she to argue with the wisdom of a higher power—or fate?

19

A RACE FOR LIFE

2:10 A.M.

They had been waiting for a signal from the desk nurse, which would allow them to see Donald. Finally it came. The woman stood, looked at them, and gave a simple nod. Margaret didn't want to go, but she had to. She was thankful that Michael and Father John were there to accompany her. She hung onto Michael's wheelchair for support until they entered the dimly lit cubicle where Donald lay on a steel cart.

It was more frightening than she imagined. His body was laid out on a stark, sterile-looking table, with a mere pad under him and only a sheet covering his legs and torso. He was not on a bed as she had expected. His head was shrouded with a towel to hide his injured face.

Bottles, cables, and tubes sprang from under the sheet. Panels of lights beeped and blinked beside him, and a respirator on the other side of the table pumped with perfect regularity, certainly more evenly than her breathing.

The slight frame was his, without a doubt. His lower arms

and hands were exposed. She bent closer. A fresh wound on his index finger marked where he had cut himself Sunday, trying to slice an editorial from the paper with one of her serrated knives. He was always clipping editorials, issues on which he either strongly agreed or disagreed. He often read the articles to her, and composed aloud the letter he should write to respond. But he never sent those letters. He guarded his privacy too closely.

She touched the small, pale feet extended beneath the sheet. Their warmth startled her. She remembered how cold her husband Paul's body had felt in his casket. She was surprised to find an electric heating pad under him. That made her feel better. She touched each toe, so perfectly formed, no corns or callouses like most people's feet. This surely was Donald. She remembered the childhood game, when his mother had recited the nursery rhyme to him. "This little piggy went to market . . ." She wiped a tear away.

"Margaret." Father John's whisper seemed to reach her through a long, narrow sound chamber. "Would you like me to anoint Donald?"

"Oh, yes." She wished for that, but I was afraid to request it. "Will that be proper?"

"Yes, certainly." He reached into the pocket of his wrinkled top coat drawing out his stole, which had been rolled into a loose ball around the holy oils and a container of holy water.

For Margaret, the words and the ritual of the anointing blunted the horror that lay beneath the cloth obscuring his face. Extreme unction, it used to be called—the last anointing. Now it was called the anointing of the sick. Just a few months ago she had congregated with other elderly and infirm at the church, where this sacrament was administered. It had been Father John who crossed her forehead with oil, asking God to ease her pains and the ravages of aging. That day she had felt the contentment now attached to the ceremony. It made the burden of the arthritis in her hips and back seem easier.

But tonight there was no comfort. This was Donald's "last anointing." Had his soul already left his body? She hoped not. She wanted his soul to have this special blessing when he faced his creator.

Father John lifted the topmost corner of the covering over Donald's head for the anointing. Margaret tried not to watch, but her mind flashed a momentary image of what must lie hidden beneath. Her stomach churned, and she forced herself to look away. She could no longer bear the pain. She grasped the handles of Michael's wheelchair and hung on, determined to weather through the short ceremony.

When it was finished, the two men helped the elderly woman back to the waiting room.

2:15 A.M.

The waiting list for liver recipients was complicated. Aren't they all? Carolyn asked herself.

At the top of the list she found Patty Goodwin's name. The liver could go to a child if her surgeon agreed. This particular transplant would require a relatively new procedure, trimming an adult liver to fit a child's cavity. Until recently, children had little chance of acquiring a cadaver liver, because it was believed that only a child's organ would fit another youngster. Yet so few children died with organs intact. Then, adult livers had been tried and found successful. Now children had a better chance at getting a transplant.

Carolyn felt reasonably certain Dr. Charles Jamison would chance to do the new surgery. However, working with Mayo Clinic's transplant program meant waiting for a Mayo-trained surgeon to do removal. That necessitated setting up for a surgeon they probably didn't know, and then standing around waiting for someone to come in and scrub. Politics, Carolyn thought with mild contempt. But she supposed it did help to have someone looking at the organ though the eyes of a surgeon trained by the transplant chief.

Patty Goodwin needs an organ—politics or no, she thought, looking at the list one last time. She placed the call, as mandated, to the chief of the liver transplant team at Mayo.

The answering service said Dr. Jamison was not on call tonight, but they would gladly notify his stand-by. However, his stand-by also would be unavailable for the next hour. Carolyn tried to be persuasive; she had to get hold of Dr. Jamison now. She came close to threatening. While she persisted, she drummed her fingers on the phone base impatiently. If Emily were here, she'd get through to Jamison immediately. If you have "doctor" in the front of your name, you always get through, she thought, scowling. She tried the number for the transplant coordinators' offices. A machine told her this was no longer a working number.

Her head began to pound. She called three coordinators she had worked with before and for whom she had home phone numbers. Surely one of them would have Dr. Jamison's inside line. One did not answer, another had an answering machine on, and the third said she no longer worked with transplants but gave her the new page number.

"Whoever's on call tonight should have Jamison's number," she volunteered. "If you strike out, call me back, I'll try to push a few buttons here."

Finally, a wasted half hour later, Carolyn connected with Meg Tyler, who promised to reach the powers-that-be.

2:20 A.M.

The charge nurse, Elaine Steiner, rushed through the door of Rudy's room trying to be calm and professional, but not succeeding.

"Mr. Popovich, they have a heart for you in Minneapolis."

Jan jolted to her feet. She must have nodded off to sleep. "I don't understand." Had she been dreaming this wondrous announcement? It took her a moment to realize that she was back in the hospital room. She looked over at Rudy, who had been medicated and seemed too groggy to hear.

"Dr. Anderson wanted to tell you himself, but we're running on a very tight timetable." The words tumbled from Elaine. "We have orders to prepare you for the trip."

Jan looked quickly at the window. "But, the storm!" The snow was gusting wildly, letting off a whistling sound.

"Dr. Anderson says he has that all arranged. Now, Mr. Popovich, I need to get your vitals."

Jan felt numb. Dr. Anderson has this blizzard "all arranged!" How?

Elaine removed the ventilator mask, put a thermometer in Rudy's mouth, and wrapped the blood pressure cuff around his arm. Rudy rallied. He sputtered and the thermometer fell from his mouth.

"Mr. Popovich, please keep your mouth shut and hold on to that thermometer. We need to get your BP right now."

Jan took Rudy's hand, causing him to turn toward her.

"Elaine said they have a heart for you," she looked at the nurse for confirmation or denial, and got neither. "In Minneapolis." Jan did not mention the inclement weather. "And Dr. Anderson will be here soon to explain everything to us." The words were only now sinking in. "Rudy, we're going to make it. We're getting you a new heart before the insurance runs out."

Rudy shook his head slowly.

Finally the nurse removed the cuff from his arm, and took the thermometer from his mouth.

"Now you can talk," she said, smiling. "And yes, it's true. You'll be leaving here in a few minutes. Just take it easy. You need to save your strength for the big trip."

"Janny, I don't understand. We're leaving tonight?"

"You bet you are," Dr. Anderson was running as he came through the door.

"How can we, doctor?" Jan remembered the storm again and her hopes took a momentary drop.

"Don't worry about a thing. There's a snowplow waiting with your ambulance downstairs. The plow and a Highway Patrol car will accompany you to the city limits, where you'll meet the county crew. There'll be more plows and sanders and Patrol cars waiting at every county line until you run out of snow. Then, you'll hightail it on to Metropolitan General. They'll be waiting for you."

As if on cue, two young men rolled an ambulance cart into the room. Immediately behind them was Julie, her uniform replaced by a thermal snowmobile suit and a stocking cap.

"Julie, have you heard the news?" Rudy called out.

"Well, why else would I be here? I intend making sure my favorite 'Raincher' gets to Minneapolis safely and on time."

Dr. Anderson rode the elevator down with them, handing Julie a small satchel. Then he gave quiet instructions, after which he gave Rudy an injection. At the Emergency Room door he took Rudy's hands in his own.

"People all over are praying for you." His voice broke just slightly. "My prayers go with theirs."

Before Rudy could respond, he was rolled out into the waiting ambulance.

Jan crawled into the back of the vehicle, past Rudy and onto a small bench seat that extended to the far corner. Julie followed her, sitting on a stool next to Rudy. As the doors closed, she immediately placed a ventilator mask on his face.

"Just to give you a few good shots of oxygen until you get settled down," she said. She also hung several bags of fluids, and restarted the IVs. As soon as she signaled through the window to the ambulance cab, they started moving. They heard the noise of the plow cranking into position. Then Jan watched a highway patrol car pull up behind them. The race for a heart had begun.

Rudy seemed to have fallen asleep from Dr. Anderson's sedative, so Julie removed the mask. His lips moved in a quiet whisper. Julie leaned forward and deciphered the message for Jan.

"Rudy says he loves you."

Jan leaned forward and tasted the salty tears as she kissed his cheek. She would not allow herself to think about the person who had died to give Rudy this chance at a new heart. Not now. She would wait until the ambulance arrived safely at the hospital and Rudy's new heart began to beat on its own.

Then she would weep for that other family.

20

MICHAEL

2:25 A.M.

When Margaret's breathing slowed to normal, Michael left
her with Father John and returned to Donald's compartment. He
could not allow his friend to lie there attended only by strangers
in these final hours. A nurse was checking monitors.

"Will I be in the way?" he asked softly.

"Not at all, sir. Take your time," the nurse said as he
wheeled in close to the gurney. "It will be a while before we will
need to disturb his body."

He watched her leave, then let loose the storm of grief
within him. The tears, the sobs, the gagging curses broke loose in
one long, throaty moan. This can't be happening. Not to Donald.
Not to me. How will I ever make it alone, without his friendship.
The torrents were finally spent, and he looked again at the form
on the table, then closed his eyes to shut out the reality.

Some considered Donald's a wasted life, Michael thought.
But they didn't really understand him. His mind was brilliant.

He was not just a friend, but a teacher, a mind-saver. Michael could not imagine what his own life might be today if Donald hadn't stimulated him and driven him to learn.

The two boys had met on the first day of second grade—a long time ago, but Michael still remembered it vividly. Perhaps they had been drawn to each other because each recognized some dread sorrow in the other. They had both lost fathers. When other boys talked about playing ball with their dads, getting help with arithmetic homework, even being hollered at by an angry father, the two seven-year-olds knew they were different from the rest.

One day a boy named James, the class bully, had taunted Michael by announcing to everyone that his "old man" had skipped town. Michael wanted to cry and run. But he stood, frozen in place, unable to breathe. The silent stares of the others paralyzed him. Then suddenly Donny walked to his side.

"His dad didn't skip town, you creep. He has to go out of town a lot on business trips. And that's where he is right now." The circled observers held their collective breaths, and Donny stood squarely, facing James as he spoke, giving the accuser a leathery, impenetrable stare.

After what seemed like hours, the bully—half a head taller than Donald—turned and walked away, muttering, "Aw, what do you know?" He never confronted either boy again. The friendship between Donald and Michael was bonded firmly in place that day. All through grade school and high school they remained close. Only those years when Donald was away at school were they separated. Again the tears came, and for the moment abated the excruciating agony.

As memories churned through his mind, Michael thought back to Donald's contemptuous resignation from the faith they shared as boys and young men. He understood Donald's sense of betrayal by a priest whom he deeply respected. But that was just one man. It was not *God* turning his back, Michael once told Donald, whose face contorted with rage.

"Oh, yes. It was. I loved your *God.* I believed Him when He spoke of peace. And how did that good *God* of yours thank me?"

Michael grasped for words. "He said, 'Blessed are the Peacemakers.'"

"Ah, yes, and I was so blessed that one of His own priests denounced me."

It was a hopeless argument. Michael tried to think of a way out. Then Donald spoke again.

"Look, Michael. We've been friends for a long time. I hope we can still be friends in the future. But there must be one condition. We will never again talk about religion. Never."

Michael had no choice but to agree. It had been so all these years. But every day Michael prayed for Donald's return to his religion. And then, it had seemed like a miracle—they began studying comparative religions. Michael would never have dared propose this inquiry. But Donald, himself, had called it a "logical, if hysterically funny, progression from astronomy. You know—stars, sky, heaven, who knows what?"

Gradually, over the few weeks of research, Donny had shifted the authorship of this project to Michael. But they both knew how it originated. Michael had watched, almost from the sidelines, as his friend delved deeper and deeper into the association of man's perceptions of God. Donny didn't know it, but Michael had already bought him a Bible. Once Donny dug into that annotated text, Michael knew he would be hooked. It was only a matter of time before they would again share the bond of faith.

But God had not waited.

2:30 A.M.

Carolyn checked her watch. This case was nerve-wracking. It was so much easier when all the recipients were nearby. Right

now, the most critical participant was trying to get through a blizzard, and she was hoping to send a liver to Rochester before the
storm spread. All the tough ones seemed to have locked-in distance factors. Must be the fates; they didn't like her. She jumped
as the phone under her elbow rang.

"Carolyn. This is Bob Anderson."

She liked doctors who acted like "real" people—not trying to distance themselves from others with their titles.

"Sorry I couldn't get back to you sooner, but there was no
time. Our man is on his way. We couldn't get a chopper off the
ground, but the Highway Patrol came through. They've arranged
everything—plows, sanding crews and patrol cars as escorts. I'd
say we're looking at three hours, if they don't run into any major
problems out there."

"Sounds terrific, Bob." She wished she *felt* "terrific"
about these logistics.

"The Highway Patrol will patch updates to you along the
way," he continued. "Has it started snowing there yet?"

"Nope. Still like a spring night according to everyone
who's been pouring into this place. The last I heard officially, the
snow stops near Hinkley, believe it or not. We checked for your
guy, and also because we have a liver going to Rochester tonight."

"Great. By the time they get out of this snow belt, they'll
be able to give you a pretty reliable time."

"The Heart Boss is standing by," she said. Everyone called
the chief heart implanter "The Heart Boss"—even his wife.
"We're sure this will be a great-looking heart."

"Thanks, Carolyn. I'm faxing the results of all tests we ran,
including those from this morning. At least that might prevent one
further delay at your end. Tell Dolan I'm counting on him." An
instant of silence. "And take good care of my man. Rudy and his
wife are very special people. Because of media reports on their
problem, they've become kind of folk heroes here. And that cre-
ates good publicity for organ donation up here—if he can make it."

They're all special, Carolyn thought. Waiting on these lists, squarely facing the potential of death every day.

Carolyn checked her watch again. We'll soon be picking up momentum here. Better give the Heart Boss our e.t.a.

21

DONALD

2:35 A.M.

The patient parking lot at Metropolitan General's Emergency Room entrance was heavily populated with cars of every make and vintage. This was center city and a typical city-supported hospital. Macrae glanced over to the entrance as she drove past. If I ever had a gun shot wound, this is where I'd want to be taken, she thought. She shivered and wondered what had made her think of that. Tonight's accident victim was killed by head injuries from some sort of accident. Same thing, ultimately, she guessed.

Henry, the white-haired night security guard came out the staff door to accompany her into the building. She smiled at him. His presence was a welcome security measure for those arriving or leaving in the late night hours. He had quickly learned who were transplant people. They were the ones who came in droves, at odd hours. Broke the monotony during night shift, he had explained.

"Evening, Macrae. Must be a big donor surgery tonight.

Lots of you folks been hurrying in here for the past half hour."

"You're right, Henry. I believe we're going to make some people very happy tonight."

"And one family will be pretty sad," he said softly.

Macrae nodded. That was the part of this job that made her uncomfortable. It wasn't her fault a man died tonight. She wanted to tell Henry that, but she knew that wasn't what he meant. Macrae always tried not to think about the donor families. She didn't know them, so it was easier to de-personalize them. Easier, but not completely doable.

Carolyn gave Macrae a welcoming pat on the shoulder.

"Popovich is on his way, and Nichols is the probable alternate. Now they're yours to worry about." She looked away, then back again, smiling. "By the way. It's nice to see you again."

"Swell. Wish I could say the same."

"That's right! You're going off to San Diego on vacation. Not tomorrow, I hope?"

"We're already into tomorrow, woman. I'm leaving Wednesday, whenever that is—if we make it through tonight."

"Well then, let's get to it."

Sometimes Macrae wished Carolyn wasn't always so darned cheerful, but it was also an endearing quality, that often relieved tension and defused short wicks.

Carolyn handed Macrae two sets of print-outs.

"As I told you, both of your men are practically in a dead heat." She turned serious, "But, because of the insurance problem with Popovich, we've edged him in ahead."

"At the office we've got his cut off date in big red letters on every calendar. This probably would be his last shot."

"Well, that's the way we called it, too—your boss and I. By the way, Jamison's on the way in. Got tired of my phone calls, I guess. Of course, it will take a while. He certainly has a long commute, even in nighttime traffic. I guess it's worth the cost of time to be able to jump into your yacht to polish off a perfect day."

Carolyn's impression of a boat skipper made them both laugh.

"By the way, he'll be using different techniques, depending upon which patient we have on the table. The donor is a relatively small man. Mr. Nichols is a better match in size, but, if it's Mr. Popovich, they'll have to compensate."

"A heterotopic?"

"Sure enough. Of course, our donor matches either of them, but Nichols still has a chance over the next few days or weeks."

"Strange about that storm, isn't it? Runs all across these states. They've got practically the entire northeast plowing, sanding, escorting, or praying. They seem optimistic, but we have no guarantees. I think you'd better check on Nichols and get him on full stand-by. Sound reasonable?"

"Sounds wonderful." Her voice was flat and, sardonic. "I love telling someone we might have a heart for him, so get ready— but then again we might decide to give it to someone else."

"It's tough," Carolyn said, "trying to play God. At least I don't have to watch the faces of the also-rans."

Macrae smiled. "What are we doing in this business, anyway?"

"Most of the time, giving out new lives—and loving the work we get to do."

As she turned to go, Macrae said, "Thanks for reminding me."

2:40 A.M.

Margaret awoke in terror, gasping and coughing. Where was she? Father John jumped, startled, his breviary flying. He scooped up the large prayer book and knelt on one knee at her side as she tried to rise from the couch. A nurse saw the incident and hurried toward them.

"Are you all right, Margaret?" The priest asked. "I think you were having a bad dream."

"Is there anything I can get you?" the nurse asked, bending toward her.

Margaret felt herself flush with embarrassment. "I think I need a rest room."

The nurse helped Margaret to her feet and steadied her before starting across the waiting room. "It's just around the corner."

Margaret nodded. "I'm all right, now. I can make it on my own."

By the time she returned to the waiting room, Father John had dozed off again, his chin on his chest, and his breviary firmly planted on his lap. Poor man, she thought. Getting dragged out in the middle of the night. We shouldn't have bothered him. But Michael was right. She had needed more assurance before making this frightening decision. But the whole business needed to be settled as quickly as possible for those poor people who were waiting.

Margaret sat down on the far end of the couch, not wanting to awaken Father John again.

She looked around the still-swarming waiting room. Who were all these people? Some had been here since she first arrived. What were they waiting for?

And she wondered about the people needing Donald's organs. How long had they been waiting? What must that kind of wait be like? For the patient, the husband or wife, just waiting? Or the mother? She remembered reading about a little boy who needed a new kidney. A church was having a big bazaar to raise money for the operation. At the time, Margaret had felt so sad for the mother and her child. She'd thought about mailing a check for the child, but she hadn't. It was just another sad story, and she'd forgotten to help. Will this make up for that forgetfulness? She hoped so.

She remembered Michael—thankful he was with Donald. Poor Donald shouldn't be left alone at a time like this. She felt a twinge of shame that she couldn't be the one to wait with him. But she'd been in there, and she couldn't bear seeing him that way. The mere thought of those towels over his head made her feel sick all over again.

What a fine man this Michael is—and she had never known him. At least Donald had him as a friend for all these years. And that was what mattered.

When Donald had returned to Minneapolis that final time, he seemed to have a considerable circle of friends. Michael, of course, was one of them. But Donald had other friends then, too. Eventually, the friends got married, relocated, or just moved on to jobs which Donald considered capitalistic.

The nurse approached Margaret with yet another form. She explained it, but Margaret was too tired to care now. She turned to Father John, who was awake again. He looked at the form and nodded. She signed the paper without comment.

"I don't know what all this signing business is about. Is there no end?" she asked him.

"I'm sure it's all routine." The priest looked at his watch. "It should be over soon." She wasn't sure what would be "over," nor did she want to ask.

"You know," she said, "Donald would be infuriated by these unending forms and all the machines and tubes hooked to his body." The priest smiled and nodded.

"He stopped trusting doctors long ago. Dentists, too, for that matter. In fact, twenty years ago his dentist said he needed surgery for gum disease or he would lose his teeth." She shook her head at the remembrance.

"So he bicycled over to the University School of Dentistry, and demanded they extract all his teeth and make him a set of false plates." She was chuckling now, though at the time she had been very upset with him.

"He was determined to be rid of what he considered the vultures of society."

"I don't know about the teeth-pulling, " Father John said, "but I think I share some of his broader viewpoint."

"He also hated all politicians, you know, and refused to vote. Some agencies, however, he had no choice but to acknowledge. He only grudgingly used banks. If he hadn't been afraid of the house burning down, he'd probably have stored his inheritance in a coffee can, hidden somewhere in his apartment." She paused to blow her nose, which seemed to be dripping constantly tonight.

"'At least they pay me for the use of my money,' he used to say, though he despised the pompousness of the money-changers—as he called them. He loved distorting the Bible for my benefit, you know." Father John patted her shoulder sympathetically.

"During the time when banks gave premiums to attract new accounts, Donald 'fixed them' by moving his accounts frequently from one bank to another to claim the newest premiums. He was partial to kitchen utensils and small appliances, which he gave as Christmas presents and sent as wedding gifts for his dwindling list of friends and relatives." She turned toward Father John again. She hadn't meant to ridicule Donald.

"He gave me a toaster when mine burned out. And one Christmas he gave me a portable mixer, because he heard me grumbling about pulling my heavy old beater out of the cupboard to mix up a package cake. He also liked luggage as a premium, though he never went anywhere to need a suitcase." Again she smiled as she spoke.

"The IRS, without question, left Donald with the highest level of bile in his throat," she said. Father John laughed aloud. They laughed together.

"Now there's something I really share with Donald," he said.

"But, still, he knew he must pay the devil his due," Margaret continued. "Paltry though that payment was. Donald was passionate about keeping the government out of his business altogether. And beyond these payments to 'Caesar,' he succeeded."

"He obviously used the public library."

She thought a moment, then slowly nodded her head at the irony. "Yes. The public library was the one governmental agency that earned his approval. They asked only that he return the books they loaned him. 'An honest enough request,' he often said."

She fell silent again, and Father John returned to his breviary.

Yes, for all his rage at forces he couldn't control, Donald was not a bad person. And Margaret would be quick to correct anyone who implied otherwise. He paid proper rent. Shoveled snow just last week, and cut the grass in summer. And he appreciated what she prepared for his dinners—with a few minor exceptions. While he didn't dislike fish, he ranted over its being served on Fridays, back when the Church required such abstinence from meat. She always served fish those days, regardless of his objections. Tears rose to her eyes.

But he was gone now. She would never cook for him again.

22

LIFE CALLS

2:55 A.M.

As soon as Meg got the message from Met Gen, she immediately placed the call to Dr. Jamison's direct line at home.

"Sorry to wake you, sir, this is Meg Tyler. Must be someone new answering your service tonight. They wouldn't let Carolyn Ames from LifeLine get through."

The expletives startled her. She couldn't fault him; this was a real screw-up by the Mayo Clinic switchboard. Nevertheless, she launched immediately into the message.

"Patty Goodwin has been matched with a donor in Minneapolis—oddly enough with a middle-aged male at Metropolitan General. But Carolyn assured me he's in remarkable physical condition, and all functions are excellent. The other coordinators say she's always been conscientious and up front in her judgements." She paused to catch her breath. Nervousness made her voice sound like a machine-gun.

"The donor is a relatively small male, who apparently lived a Spartan life. No indication of any abuse of the body—no drugs or alcohol. Exceptional muscle tone."

"I think we should take it," Jamison interrupted. "But I want one of our people to harvest and evaluate the organ. You have the list of our people?"

"Yes, sir, at the hospital. I'm still at home, but it will only take me a few minutes to get dressed and over to the office."

"Confirm it with Met Gen. And when you find a surgeon available, have 'em call me. I'd like to have some specific observations. Oh, if you can't find anyone up there, call me back and we'll send a team."

"And the Goodwins?"

"Might as well hold off until we get more information. We have a potential of eight hours after excision."

"Sounds fine, sir. Maybe I can take a little snooze at the hospital." She hoped she sounded jovial, not whiny. She tried to sound human around Dr. Jamison, but she was awestruck whenever she talked to him. She had observed him at the hospital for years, never dreaming she would one day be working with him—or, more correctly, for him.

"Good idea," he said. "That way we don't have to pay you time and a half this week." She was relieved to hear the tease in his voice. "Tell Carolyn we want ongoing reports, so we can gauge when to assemble."

So much for napping, Meg thought, not minding a bit.

The parking ramp was nearly empty when she arrived at Mercy Hospital. She chose a prime spot, next to the elevator shaft.

"There have to be some perks for the crazy hours of this job," she muttered.

3:00 A.M.

Carolyn's call hit Nancy Martinez with strongly ambivalent emotions. Katherine Lonsdale had been at the top of the recipient list for several weeks, and now, finally, there was a matching kidney available for her. Of course, Nancy wanted Katherine to get that organ, but she was also afraid it might be too late for her.

"Who's the donor," Nancy asked, more as a moment's stall for time to think.

"A forty-something male." Sounded a little old to Nancy, but beggars can't be choosers. "Riding his bicycle." That struck a promising chord—a physically active man, even in winter. "Hit head on with a truck. All injuries cranial."

"Good shape otherwise?"

"Mint condition."

"How's the match?"

"Looks like a five."

That did it. A five out of six antigen match between donor's and recipient's blood was excellent. Without a good match, antigens, which coat the surface of every blood cell, could raise havoc with a transplanted organ. The more donor antigens matching the recipient's, the less likely the chance that a recipient's immune system would slough off the new, invading organ. The only perfect matches, of course, were identical twins, who inherit the same six antigens, three from each parent, when the fertilized egg is split. They didn't need any anti-rejection drugs, either. Everybody should have an identical twin, Nancy thought. Katherine Lonsdale, however, did not even have close matches in her family. A cadaver organ was her only hope. And for this situation, the five match was very good.

"Katherine's not only in an extremely weakened physical condition, but her mental state is also bad. I'm not really sure if she has the will to live anymore." Nancy wished she could take back the words the instant she'd said them.

"I think I'd give up, too, after all she's been through."

"Hey, Carolyn, this is not a value judgement. I just want to make sure that if we give her this new kidney, she will have the determination to survive." But Nancy knew it really was a value judgement, and that troubled her.

"I understand, really. And it's your call."

"Actually it's Mike Sciaretta's call. He's the designated surgeon on this one, so I go with whatever he says." Nancy wondered why she was being so defensive tonight. Still half asleep, probably.

"How soon can you get back to me?"

"Soon. I'll get a preliminary inclination from Sciaretta, then call you. If that's a go, I'll arrange to meet the husband at Greenwood for a final look-see. I suspect Sciaretta may want to be in on that meeting, too. And that means maybe two hours before we have a definite response. Is that all right?"

"Sounds fine. We'll have plenty of time on a kidney to go for an alternate, if one is needed."

"By the way, who's on top for the other kidney?"

"One of Mimi's people. They'll do the work at Memorial Central."

"Just checking. You know I have a nice long list sitting on my desk. So any time you need another recipient, just holler."

"Don't get greedy, girl. I'm not Santa Claus."

Perhaps not, Nancy thought, but each viable organ Carolyn had sent her way was a gift without measure.

Actually she could have anticipated Mike Sciaretta's response.

"I want Katherine to get this kidney. No "ifs," period."

Of course, he was right. However, Nancy knew he also had another, perhaps stronger agenda for this kidney transplant. Katherine had been skidding downward physically and emotionally over the past weeks. No well-matched kidneys had appeared for her. To better prepare her for a wider range of potential matches, Mike had initiated a controversial preparatory procedure. He began a series of non-related blood transfusions, one pint every other day over the past two weeks. He had explained it to Mr. Lonsdale as a stabilizing treatment, which it could well be. However, the transfusions had a secondary—perhaps even a primary—goal of modulating Katherine's immune system by confusing it with new blood antigens, enabling her body to be less hostile to a foreign organ.

"This," he had explained to Nancy, "could allow the successful transplantation of an organ with a less than ideal match."

But a five-match was just that much better. Only time would tell if the transfusions did, indeed, help the body accept the transplanted kidney—requiring, perhaps, lower dosages of Prednisone and Cyclosporine.

Mike, also as expected, did want to see Katherine at Greenwood. She had been scheduled for a move to Metropolitan General the following morning—after her baby was discharged. Mike would check her tonight.

However, his assurance that he could be there in an hour stretched credibility beyond the bounds of reality. These gentlemen farmers tended to underplay the inconvenience of country living. Perhaps they set these impossible time targets so that everyone would be in place when the master sauntered in. Doctors must never be kept waiting. She had long ago learned how many minutes there were in one of Mike's hours—closer to ninety.

In any case, it was time to call Bob Lonsdale.

23

A RUN FOR HOPE

3:05 A.M.

The thick snow was falling heavily, but they drove on. The ice beneath them made the ambulance stop and start every few minutes. As the interstate rounded the crest of the long hill leading out of Duluth, Jan strained to look back at the normally splendid view of the city and harbor lights. Only a soft, grey flush glowing through the nearly opaque swirls of snow gave any hint that civilization lay behind them. Several episodes of spinning wheels and fishtailing occurred as the driver battled the long, icy climb to the top. Several times, the driver jammed on the brake, slowing the vehicle so suddenly that things fell in a heap around her. Jan breathed easier when she finally felt the ambulance level off.

They stopped at Proctor, the first town along the freeway. The driver got out of the car; the other attendant opened the chamber window and asked.

"All right?"

Julie gave him a thumbs-up.

"Sorry about the shimmying on the hill," he said. "It was pretty slick in places. They're closing the highway now that we're through."

The long hill was often closed in bad storms. The thought of someone else needing to leave the city tonight troubled Jan. She had never thought twice in the past about anyone's life depending upon getting out. The closeness of their near-miss spawned cold chills.

"We're picking up a new plow crew here at Proctor," the attendant said. "We'll meet a sanding truck a few miles ahead. Then we change crews again at Moose Lake." His smile was comforting.

Rudy called out in a hoarse voice. Julie interpreted. "He wants to know why we have stopped and to say we have to keep going."

The attendant cupped his hands around his mouth to be heard.

"Don't worry, Mr. Popovich; you're on top priority. The Highway Patrol is determined to get you to Minneapolis—and on time—even if they have to hand shovel us all the way."

Rudy again tried to speak. Julie transmitted the message. "He says that's fine, as long as he doesn't have to get out there and shovel."

"I don't think we have to worry on that score," the attendant said.

Jan and Julie stretched their stiff backs and leg muscles.

"I'm sorry, ladies, that we don't have comfortable seating for this long a trip. If either of you would like to trade places, I'd be glad to come back there."

Both spoke at once. "No, thanks."

"This is fine, really it is," Jan added.

The driver's door opened and they heard voices outside. He leaned back into the cab.

"Just got a report from the highway patrol car," he said. "The snow lets up at Hinkley."

"Wonderful," everyone said in unison.

The attendant closed the window between them. The driver knocked his boots against the running board, kicking off the caked snow. He slammed the door shut, and they were on the way again.

Jan tried to resettle herself on her perch. Every stiff muscle—as well as her sore bottom—was worth it if they made it to Minneapolis in time.

Eventually they drove out of the snow. The plows and sanders turned back, but a highway patrol car continued with them.

Jan fully relaxed for the first time since leaving the hospital. She had tried not to worry about the snow, but such concerns were learned in childhood. Winter storms could always turn treacherous. But it should be smooth sailing from here. She laid her head back into the corner of the vehicle. Before she dozed off, she resolved not to look at her watch again until they were there.

That resolution would be broken several times during the remaining miles.

3:10 A.M.

After leaving Kate at the hospital, Bob had dropped into bed, exhausted. Sleep entombed him. Then, with bullet-like ferocity, a thought shot through his unconsciousness, bringing him to his feet in a jungle sweat.

In the cool air of the bedroom, Bob Lonsdale shivered from the wetness that saturated his body. His pajamas felt drenched. Still wearing them, he stepped into the shower, begging the full blast of hot water to cleanse the terror that had pressed against his chest.

He shed the wet pajamas and wrapped himself in a full-length, hooded robe. In the kitchen, he poured a brandy, thought about tomorrow, then poured it back into the bottle, choosing instead a Perrier. It was three in the morning. He couldn't remember what time he had turned off the bedside lamp.

He walked into the dark living room to the wall of lakeview windows that brought the world to his feet. The moon highlighted the ridges and rims of the frozen lake. Now and then, a car blipped through the pattern of light on the street below. A north wind blew pages of newspapers across the lake shore jogging trail, which was still used by the most dogged of runners.

The night looked colder than when he had come home. He touched the glass; it seemed cooler.

As always, the view comforted Bob.

What had awakened him? A dream? About his wife, Kate? Whatever it was, it was gone, and he was thankful.

Tomorrow he would be bringing his baby daughter, Kathleen, home. He looked back over his shoulder at the broad openness they had loved about this condo. He wished Kate were home. How many nights had they stood here together looking down at the lake? How many nights had they fallen asleep together on the long white sectional opposite the windows, their bodies spooned, warm flesh against warm flesh? He wished they could have this one last night together—alone. From tomorrow on, their days and nights would be inexorably changed. They would be a family—if his wife survived. Their baby Kathleen was two months old, but this was the first time he had ever thought of her as a real part of their lives.

A thought jolted him. What if the nurses he'd hired to take care of the baby didn't show up tomorrow or other days? He paced anxiously back and forth in front of the window, the moonlight providing a softly-lit track. Okay, he told himself, get a handle on this now. He would ask the agency about lining up short-notice substitutes. Surely that was a common problem. If that didn't work, he'd just have to take leave from his practice for a while, and stay home. No problem.

Everyone at the office was very supportive. Besides, Kate won't be spending the rest of her life in the hospital. At least he hoped not. He took a deep drink of the cold water and sat down on the sofa, staring, yet not seeing the silent world that spread across the lake.

Poor little Kathleen. What had all these weeks in the hospital been like for her? What was she coming home to? Three nurses a day. Always a different pair of arms holding her. And, in between, he was supposed to bond with her when he knew nothing about caring for any child, let alone this tiny infant. For all her progress, she still weighed under six pounds, less than most newborns.

He should get some sleep, but he was wide awake. He went into the bedroom. The bed was soaked with his perspiration. He took the blanket out to the sofa and wrapped himself in it. The maid would change the bedding tomorrow anyway. He felt ready for sleep now.

The phone's ring startled him. His heart pounded again. What was wrong? Was it Kate or Kathleen? He fumbled in the darkness for the phone.

"Yes?" He tried to soften his breathless shout.

"Mr. Lonsdale, this is Nancy Ramirez from the Metropolitan General's transplant center. I'm sorry to have awakened you at this hour."

Bob was trying to follow her words. But he had to switch gears. "I'm sorry, who did you say you were?"

"Nancy Ramirez, kidney coordinator at the Metropolitan General transplant center. We met on one of my visits to your wife—when she was placed on the kidney waiting list."

"Oh, yes, now I remember."

"Well, Mr. Lonsdale, I just got word that we have a kidney available tonight, which is an excellent match for Katherine."

Bob's heart seemed to stop. "You have a kidney for Kate?"

"Yes, a well-matched kidney. However, there is one small problem I'd like to talk over with you." Bob's emotions were skidding out of control. "As I've been visiting your wife over the past few weeks, I've been disturbed by her deepening depression."

"Yes, she has been depressed. Sometimes I think she's lost all hope."

"Depression is not uncommon for patients waiting for transplant organs. Our staff psychiatrist evaluated her two weeks ago, but his findings were inconclusive."

"You had a psychiatrist see Kate?" Bob did not like his wife being turned over to a shrink when she was so ill.

"It's standard procedure, Mr. Lonsdale. We like all potential organ recipients to have a psychiatric evaluation. We like to be sure that anyone we give an organ to is mentally stable enough to commit to a lifetime of recovery after the surgery. With her medical conditions, we didn't want to use anti-depressant medications. We could only hope that she could work herself through this despondency. Katherine was to have another evaluation tomorrow. But, of course, we can't wait for that now. How about you, Mr. Lonsdale? Please be honest. Do you believe your wife has the drive to get well?"

For a split second he doubted. But he knew Kate.

"Yes. I feel certain that once she hears the news, she'll be back in the game fighting for her life."

"All right, Mr. Lonsdale, we'll go for it. Would you like to be there when we tell her? It's helpful for a family member to be present. Four ears are better than two."

"Yes, indeed. I'll be there in a half hour."

"Don't break the speed limit, Mr. Lonsdale. Time counts, but not as much as safety. I have a few more phone calls to make before I leave for Greenwood. We'll be transferring your wife to Metropolitan General, so I have a number of arrangements to make at both hospitals. Nothing to worry about, I assure you. Normally we'd have automatically transferred her over when your baby was released. But we tried to make it a little easier for you. But now we can go ahead with the transfer.

"Also, Dr. Sciaretta, who will be doing her surgery, wants to see her before she's moved. Just to be sure she's stabilized for this surgery. He is at his farm down Interstate 35, near New Prague. So it's going to take him an hour to get in. And we find it's best if we all, including you, go into the patient's room together. It will be a lot less confusing for Mrs. Lonsdale."

"That means if I get there first, I should wait for you?"

"If you don't mind."

"No, I want this to go by the book."

"Okay, Mr. Lonsdale, but I'd better warn you that it rarely happens that we 'go by the book.' There are just too many variables." He heard a smile in her voice. It was comforting.

"At any rate, when I first get to Greenwood, I'll arrange for her transferral and line up an ambulance for the move. I think we're looking at an hour minimum from now."

"Ms. Ramirez, I think it would be very good for Kate to have her old friend, Dr. Ben Coslow there, too—either when she is told, or for the surgery. I am sure he'd want to know, anyhow. May I call him?"

"That's a great idea, but why don't you let me call him? You probably have a long enough list right now, what with plans to bring little Kathleen home tomorrow."

"I hadn't thought about that. When would Kate's surgery be performed?"

"Well, they're about ready here at Met Gen to begin harvesting the organs. Time is a sparse commodity for the heart and liver, but kidneys are the last removed and can actually be held for a couple of days. However, we're very anxious to get one of these fine kidneys neatly planted into your wife as soon as possible. They already have an operating room reserved for us, but there's set-up time. I'd say not before eight o'clock. I'll plan to meet you at Glenwood in an hour and a quarter. By then I may have a better fix on surgery time, also. Okay?"

"Oh, yes. That's very okay."

Bob hung up the phone. He wanted to jump, shout, yell. The sense of excitement overwhelmed him. But shards of fear stabbed at his joy. "Come on, man, get hold of yourself," he told the bathroom mirror. "This is it. This is what you've been waiting for."

Still in his robe, he started back to the kitchen. He needed a bump of caffeine. He hated instant, but there wasn't time now to brew a pot—a skill he'd finally mastered over the past few months. In the hallway, he caught sight of the wall of family pictures. Kate's parents. He had to call them.

He was too excited and nervous to be logical or direct. Above the nervous pounding of his heart, he heard himself saying the words: "I'd be very happy to have you both come." For his mother-in-law's benefit, he added, "I thought you might like to be here during Kathleen's first week or so at home. We'll have the nurses, so you'll be free to spend time with Kate, too."

She sounded pleased—a far more compassionate Barbara than the one he'd known over the years. Why hadn't it occurred to him that she and George were as worried as he was over Kate and Kathleen? Even before this illness, he and the Landers had never had a real chance to get acquainted. Perhaps they had always worried about Kate and this stranger she had married.

"It would be wonderful for Kathleen, Barbara. Would you like to come straight to the hospital tomorrow? Good. We'll be moving Kate tonight to Metropolitan General Medical Center for the surgery. Right downtown off Interstate thirty-five. You can ask at the main desk for directions to the transplant center. I'll be there."

He was struggling to keep his emotions in check.

"Thanks, Barbara. Thank you so much."

What an extraordinary time this would be. Kate was going to get well!

She had to.

24

LISTS

3:30 A.M.

As she waited for further word, Carolyn studied the pages
of computer printout, once more reading over the four recipient
files, keeping in mind that kidneys were the organs with the
longest durability. Both top kidney contenders were fairly close
by, but a disturbing thought suddenly gave her concern.
Something was wrong—and it had to do with the logistics and
time of the liver transplant.

If Mr. Popovich made it in, he might be too late. The
donor heart had a short availability and no one knew for certain
what its exact condition was. It had to be in full view before the
first incision was made on Mr. Popovich. And the liver harvesting
had to be done immediately after the heart. Back on the phone—
to Rochester.

"Meg, this is Carolyn again. Have your people decided yet
on whether or not you want our liver?

"You didn't get my message?" Meg replied agitatedly. "I
called the number I had for you nearly a half hour ago, and left

a message. Obviously, you didn't get it. Yes. Dr. Jamison definitely wants this liver."

"Fine." Carolyn replied without much enthusiasm. Actually, she had hoped that they'd turn it down.

"Do you have someone heading in for the removal?"

"No, I've been making calls, but haven't connected yet. I'll keep trying. If I can't reach anyone, we'll send a team up from here to do the harvesting."

"Sorry, Meg. There's not enough time. We have a Status-One heart recipient coming through a blizzard. We expect him in approximately two hours. It's a long story, but it's now or never for this man. He must get this heart tonight before his insurance runs out—which means, we must have our donor open and the heart retrieved in two hours. The liver has to go next. That can only work if you find a surgeon available up here. It's too tight for your team to collect in Rochester and get to us in time."

"Oh, dear." It was more of a gasp. Tonight was Meg Tyler's solo debut. Heck of a time to start, Carolyn thought, biting her lip and pausing for a moment.

"Meg, I know this is a tough one. Jamison has a well-known policy about harvesting, but, if it's down to the wire, Tom Hartung, who did the cranial surgery, is still here. He's a top trauma man. If Jamison wants him to do the work, he has to know very soon so that he can pull his team together. I don't mean for this to sound like a threat, but we have to be assured the patient gets this organ when its viable. The waiting list is too long. It's just the reality here. We'll start faxing all the donor's records as soon as we hear from you. But It has to be soon."

An uneasy silence came over the wire, then Meg replied softly but firmly.

"I'll call Dr. Jamison right away, and get back to you in a few minutes."

Meg sounded like the wind had just been knocked out of her, Carolyn thought. This is a tough business she has gotten into, and tonight would be a difficult initiation. She hoped Meg could hold it together.

3:35 A.M.

Meg had already called five surgeons on the list. All unavailable. Two remote possibilities remained. She had been forewarned by her predecessor that surgeons with established practices no longer appreciated "go-fer" calls in the middle of the night—and it was turning out to be true.

Now Carolyn had delivered new complications. Meg dreaded making the next phone call to Jamison. She never liked giving anyone bad news. Before she called, she would check Patty's condition.

Maureen, the charge nurse, answered the phone.

"She's extremely critical. She may not make it beyond tonight. I was just going to call her parents. I don't suppose you have any good news for us, do you?"

"A slight possibility." She didn't want to build false hope. "If you can, hold off on her parents until I reach Dr. Jamison again. I'll be back with you one way or the other within ten minutes."

Meg paused before punching the last digit of Dr. Jamison's phone number. He'd be expecting word from the designated "Mayo Man" in Minneapolis. She took a deep breath and tapped the final button.

"This is Meg again, sir. I tried five people from the list— all unavailable tonight. I have a couple more to try, but Gena told me these surgeons were no longer happy with our emergency calls. *And*, we have other problems—here and in Minneapolis."

"What kind of problems?" His terseness was unsettling.

"They've got a heart recipient coming in and he's expected in two hours. They have to give him top priority—something about his insurance running out. It boils down to their having to start on the donor before we can get a team up there."

"Damn, I wanted that liver, but I wanted one of our people there to eye-ball it for me. You've heard, no doubt, how I feel about getting a firsthand account of what we're facing."

"I know that, sir, and so does Carolyn Ames. However, as I said, we now have a problem here, too. I just talked to ICU. Patty's extremely critical. Maureen was about to call her parents."

Jamison was silent for a moment.

"Who handled the donor's original surgery at Met Gen?"

"Carolyn specifically mentioned him, a Dr. Thomas Hartung."

"I've heard of him. He's supposed to be a fine trauma surgeon, even if he isn't one of ours." Meg caught the quip, the standard Rochester bias which many still held dear to their hearts. She was relieved by the change in his tone.

"He must have considerable experience with harvesting organs."

"Carolyn intimated that he was very capable. And she said she'd fax the donor's records if that would help us."

More silence. Meg felt another twinge of nervousness. Luckily, Jamison was a pragmatic man.

"Is Hartung still suited for surgery?"

"Carolyn indicated that he was, but he does have to round up his team people."

"Do we have an alternate recipient here, just in case? Once we bring the liver here, there won't be time for another transport. And I don't want any viable organs going to waste"

"Yes, sir, I checked our list, and we do have at least two other prospects.

"Very well, let's take it. This little girl deserves the best shot we can give her." Meg virtually jumped off the floor with excitement.

"When you talk to Met Gen, tell them we want a charter

flight. I want that organ here as soon as possible—to see it and work on a formula for down-sizing. Order a plane or a chopper from here, unless they have one they recommend. Let me know the timing. Oh, yes, ask Hartung to call me before he starts. I'd like some general observations, as well as venous measurements, I want everything ready on this end."

"Got it," Meg said—more to slow down the note-taking than to respond. "Should I call the Goodwins now?"

"Check with Maureen, and have her put someone at Patty's side from this point on. Let the Goodwins sleep if Patty is holding. They're going to have a long wait ahead of them once we start. We can at least get the timing straight first. Call me when you have . . . Oh, what the hell, I'm wide awake now. I'm coming in. I'll probably be there before Hartung gets in gear. Give him my page number."

A shiver of exhilaration shot up Meg's back.

"Give Met Gen the go-ahead and have the transportation arranged," Jamison continued. "Call the Goodwins when you get a fix on time. No rush, but I will want to talk to them beforehand about this procedure. We'll put out the call for the surgical team and support personnel after I get there. And put Andy Smith on your list for later calls. He's got a real attachment to that child. And I'd like her to see his face before she goes under."

"You bet. He'll certainly want to be here."

The surgical wing was quiet tonight—for now, at least. Meg liked it this way. During the day the place was like a railroad station, people moving in every direction, voices, clatter, phones ringing, carts with patients lined up along the hallways. Amidst the chaos, coordinators scheduled transplants, arranged for operating rooms and surgical teams, got patients prepped and saw that families had time for last minute visits.

But tonight, her first time alone, everything seemed peaceful. She could work undistracted, making absolutely sure everything was on line before she started rousing people all over Rochester. Now there was time to check every step, every test result—which was a blessing. She had been looking forward to this night since she first dreamed of being a coordinator. Tonight was her first time to go it alone. She had no back-up—she had to do it right.

She arranged for surgery in the main OR theater. News spread quickly at the hospital. Only a few weeks ago, Dr. Jamison had issued a paper outlining the new procedures for using an adult organ, trimmed and fitted to the correct size for transplantation into children. The gallery would fill quickly when word got out that an eight-year-old was to receive the liver of a middle-aged man. New procedures always heightened interest.

Meg waited impatiently at the fax machine for the donor's charts Carolyn was sending. At least Jamison would have all the donor data, in black and white, well ahead of surgery. This was no time for a screw-up.

25

COUNTDOWN

3:45 A.M.

"Hey, Tom! Enough of this lally-gagging."

A wide grin accompanied Carolyn Ames's announcement as she came into the lounge area.

"I have just sold your services to Mayo—for a liver."

"Well, I'll be darned. What happened?"

"I'm a good salesperson. Actually, we're running out of time, and so is Mayo. Apparently they have a little girl who badly needs this liver. Also, your fragile heart recipient is en route."

"You don't miss a thing do you?"

"I collect scraps of dialogue—like some people collect rubber bands or aluminum foil."

"Why am I not surprised?" he said, one eyebrow cocked in a mock cynicism.

"Have you set a time yet with Dolan?"

"Nope. That's my next call."

Hartung turned to his staff, strewn about comfortably in the lounge.

"Okay, gang, the slave-driver's sending us back to the trenches. Becky, we'll be following the Heart Boss—extracting a liver for Mayo Clinic, mind you." He waited for her appropriate reaction, which she conveyed by giving him a wink.

"We won't need any more people to do the opening, but we'll need the rest of the team for the liver. Will you send the word out, please?"

Becky snapped to attention and saluted. "Will do."

He glanced from her to Carolyn, shaking his head.

"I'm beginning to understand poor ol' Rodney Dangerfield." Both women laughed as they turned to go. Then Carolyn turned back, once more the professional.

"Oh, yes—Dr. Jamison wants you to call him before you start. General condition and measurements," Meg said. She handed Hartung a memo with the number, and returned to the main desk.

Max had arrived. That was a load off her mind. Max had been an orderly when Carolyn discovered him. He had an uncanny way of seeing what needed to be done and doing it. He was exactly the kind of person Carolyn had been hoping to find. So she got Emily to push the right buttons to get him assigned to the transplant center, with the title of "Transplant Technician," which could be translated into a pay raise—as well as a little more dignity for Max. His was a welcome face tonight.

After a moment of welcome, she briefed him on the medical and transportation problems for the night.

"Here it is, Max. Mayo wants a charter. They'll sign for it. Keep in close contact with the weather service. A charter could be touchy if that storm moves this way. Keep tight with Meg Tyler and have someone here designated to reconfirm with her the minute you're out the door with the Igloo cooler." She sighed. "I guess that's it for now."

Max, unflappable as ever, smiled patiently. She envied him that quality. And she loved him for the ballast he provided, and the fact that he was always 100 percent reliable.

$\mathcal{L}ife\mathcal{L}ine$

The waiting room crowd was thinning out. Some had left with smiles of relief, others in sorrow. When Margaret left she would be among the latter. She could still not believe this monstrous nightmare was really happening. Why? Why? Oh god, not my Donald.

Another thought pounced upon her. She must arrange his burial. Most of her savings had been earmarked for her own funeral expenses. Now she would have to use that money to bury Donald, who had been like a son to her.

A moment's panic: Who will bury me? I was the one who was supposed to die first. I had explained all that to him. He had scoffed at talk of death and burial and told her not to worry; he'd dig a hole in the back yard for her. Still she knew he would have followed her wishes and arranged a proper interment.

She had understood him, at least most of the time. His sarcasm had been a way of covering his fears and uncertainties. He was a man of contradictions. All that needling talk, and yet gentle Donald could not kill even a bothersome fly or mosquito that followed him into the house. With great patience he would steer the smallest insect back to freedom.

Michael was right. Donald would approve of his organs saving others' lives. Margaret tried to take some satisfaction from the gift, but she felt awash, smothered, remembering Donald's sensitive side he tried so belligerently to hide, even from her. As immune to others as he wished to appear, he did not succeed most of the time—most particularly the day *they* had come.

Her mind spun backwards.

≈

While many only-children expressed loneliness at not having brothers or sisters, Donald enjoyed his singular status in the family. At the age of seven, he confidently assumed his role as core of his widowed mother's life. Margaret and Paul were thrilled to have him as part of their family. Of course, when he began his university years—after both Paul and Marie were dead—he was gone most of the time. By his visits, letters, and phone calls always kept him close to her.

By the time Donald finally came back, only his aunt remained for him. Though he struggled to maintain his independence, she saw his hunger for love and acceptance. Margaret had never found it easy to show emotion, either, but, in time she realized that whatever nonsense he spoke—however many locks he placed on his doors—he knew she cared deeply about him. And there was no doubt in her mind that he felt the same for her.

They lived relatively separate lives. Their few relatives and friends gave them whatever outside fulfillment they needed as their lives moved in a set of barely overlapping circles. She was content, and was reasonably certain he was, too.

Then, not long after he'd come home, *they* arrived.

Two women—blondish with piquant faces, strangely like Donald's—were at the door when she answered the bell. They asked if she knew the whereabouts of a Donald Mills. This sounded ominous. She asked them to wait. Her hand trembled as she knocked twice on his door, another code between them. They all listened to his footsteps descending on the stairs. When he opened his door, she nodded toward the women and went into her apartment and back to the kitchen so she would not be tempted to eavesdrop. But her pulse pounded in her ears.

Some time later, Donald appeared, ghostly white, standing at the kitchen door, asking her to come into the living room. He shifted from one foot to the other, like a nervous child facing the principal after school, while she washed and wiped her hands.

The women stood as she entered; both towered over Donald and Elizabeth.

"These women say they are my half-sisters." His face was stoic; his voice flat and steady.

This was utter nonsense, she thought, but she saw that

Donald believed them. She looked from him to each woman and back again. Then one of them spoke.

"My name is Francis Mills, and this is my half-sister Helen Curtin. We're both from the Los Angeles area. We've recently discovered that our father appears to have led three separate, sequential lives—with three different women—and produced, along the way, a child by each wife."

This was a bold-faced lie. Marie would certainly have told Margaret if this were true. Besides, she wouldn't have married a man who had already been married before. Why, their wedding was in a Catholic church, for heaven's sake.

Donald stared at the floor, still shifting his feet. The woman continued.

"I'm the second child— by the second wife. When I was about seventeen, I visited my father and Donald's mother in New York. This was before he was born, of course," she said, nodding toward Donald.

"I've just shown Donald this picture." She handed the old photo to Margaret. It was Marie and Harry, standing on either side of a girl—a girl of about seventeen. Marie was smiling, but it was a different expression than Margaret had ever seen on Marie's face—as if two halves of different photographs had been fused together. The lower portion of her face smiled, but in the upper half, she seemed almost to be crying. That must have been when she learned of the lie Harry was living. Margaret also noted that Marie appeared to be in the middle months of pregnancy.

Margaret handed back the picture and the other woman took up the chronology.

"Some years ago, after my parents were killed in an automobile crash, I began looking into my family tree. I pulled out an old box of my parents' papers and discovered that the man I knew as my father was, in fact, my step-father. In that box, I found my birth certificate and my mother's earlier divorce decree from a Harry Mills. I was shocked, but I had to continue searching. Los Angeles was a smaller town then. Old phone books and city directories led me to the neighborhood where Helen grew up—and finally to Helen. Her recollections of that visit out east took us to New York and the company where our father had worked. The company's old stock and insurance records listed another offspring, a son, Donald, and that information brought us to Minneapolis. It's incredible that he is still at this address. We weren't sure we'd ever find him."

Donald did not seem to react. But Margaret felt his shock, the pain of this bewildering betrayal by both his parents. He seemed to be curling into himself.

Margaret remembered going to kitchen to make coffee—anything to get out of that room! When she returned, Donald was just closing the door behind them. He said nothing, but his face was ashen when he went up to his apartment. He did not come down that night for dinner. Margaret wanted to go up and comfort him, reassure him that he still had his place in her love. But she wasn't good at that sort of thing. She had no words. In the waste basket next to her chair she saw the photo, torn into four pieces. She found a business card lying on the coffee table. Without reading beyond the name, Helen Curtin placed it in the drawer of her telephone stand.

The next evening Donald came down for dinner. He ate in silence. The subject of his half-sisters was never again mentioned between them. It was days before he began to speak or leave the house. She never knew what Donald had said to the women, but she didn't believe there had been any further contact.

ƨ

Father John awoke with a startled expression.

"I'm sorry, I must have dozed off." She wished he didn't have to lose this night's sleep.

He stood up and rearranged his rumpled clothing.

"You should try to get some sleep, Margaret."

"I'll have plenty time for that later," she said. "I've been thinking; Donald had sisters, you know, half-sisters."

"Yes, you told me about that once. I was thinking of them a while ago. I couldn't remember where they lived."

"California. I have one's business card at home. I don't know why I kept it. For this, I suppose."

There was silence again.

"Margaret, does Donald have a will?"

"Donald? Heavens, no—at least I don't think so. He would never have allowed a lawyer to meddle in his affairs. Besides, he thought he was going to live forever."

"Why don't you let me notify the sisters?"

She was relieved.

"I'll stop in when I take you home and pick up the card." She nodded. "And Margaret, don't worry about his funeral. If he has bank accounts, there's money there for that. And also there should be money from the truck driver's insurance."

Funny, she hadn't thought of that. She was relieved.

Father John thought a moment.

"I don't suppose he had health insurance."

"I used to work in an insurance office; so I always carried health insurance. But he said he didn't need doctors, that he could make himself well if he got sick. And he always did. But this time, he can't."

"Don't worry about the medical bills, either. The driver's insurance will cover that, too."

There was quiet again as both stared into the emptiness.

"I suppose the sisters will get whatever money he has." Her words barely hinted at a question.

"I don't know. You'll need a lawyer to tell you that. But, unless he had a will, it is a possibility." He patted her hand.

She looked at the priest and smiled.

"I guess now he's going to have lawyers and the govern- ment—and those sisters—meddling in his affairs after all."

"That is ironic, isn't it? But Margaret, you mustn't worry

about any of that. All the hospital and funeral costs will be paid before anyone gets a nickel of his money."

She looked at him, puzzled.

"I thought that young woman said the people who got his organs paid all the costs."

"All the costs since he has been declared brain-dead." As she winced at the words, he regretted using the term.

"But some of the costs will be his—charged to his estate. The ambulance, the first surgery, those kinds of things. But Margaret, please don't worry about that now. Put that all out of your mind. A lawyer will take care of those things later."

Margaret's head pounded. There was too much happening, too much to think about, too many decisions to make. Maybe Father John was right, she should put this all out of her mind. But what was there to put back into her mind to replace it? There was nothing left.

26

ALMOST

Roger Burrows had moved down the stairs From the etagere he removed his father's old service revolver, Roger's one momento of the old fella's police career. Roger had always kept it loaded, though he never knew why. Now he knew.

Slowly, he positioned the barrel at his left temple. He could hear voices on the television set in the living room. Suddenly, a strange beeping noise broke over the other sounds.

Almost by instinct, as if suspecting a burglar, he got up, gun in hand, and made his way slowly to the archway of the living room. The pager was sitting on the table. And it was beeping.

Roger froze. He was supposed to keep that pager with him at all times, but he'd forgotten it in his anguish. How long had it been sounding? He had an instant vision of his kidney going to someone else. Putting down the gun, he leaped to the box and turned it off. Quickly, he dialed the phone number posted on the back.

"This is Roger Burrows."

"Yes, Roger. This is Mimi at Memorial Central." He

recognized her without her telling him. The urgency in her voice told him this was no ordinary call.

"I was beginning to worry that you weren't getting our page. I have great news for you. We've just gotten word from the organ procurement folks. It looks like we have a kidney that's a really good match for you."

Again Roger froze. What had she said? His heart pounded so loudly he couldn't hear.

"Hey, Roger. Are you there?"

"Yes. I'm here. You found a kidney for me? Already? Tonight? I can't believe it."

"Well, it's actually morning now, but that's just a technicality. Tell me, are you feeling all right? Have any cold or flu symptoms cropped up since you were here? No crap now. Don't try to con me."

"Oh, yes, I mean no, I'm feeling fine." Actually he was sweating so much that he thought he might pass out.

"Is you wife there?"

"No. Not at the moment."

"Roger, it's almost four in the morning. Where is she—at the moment?"

He wasn't sure they would understand. He had never told them that she traveled a lot—or that she needed to keep working for his insurance.

"She's in Atlanta on business."

"Atlanta. Okay, Roger. Are you up to taking a cab over here, or should I send an ambulance for you?"

"No. I'm fine. I'll call a cab. When do you want me there?"

"As soon as you've made the necessary arrangements at home."

"I'm on my way."

The line went dead, but Roger hung onto his phone. He was certain the "necessary arrangements" meant calling Martha. He considered the idea. No, that was pointless. There was no way

Martha could get here now, and there was nothing she could do—but worry. And she already had enough of that. No, Martha might as well get a good night's sleep.

His hands shook as he laid the phone in its cradle. His mind and stomach were both doing gymnastics. He sat down. He couldn't seem to move. He should do something, but what?

Then the thought came to him. He had almost missed the call! Almost missed another chance at life. He would be dead now if it weren't for this remarkable little gizmo. He fondled the pager for a moment.

Okay, old man. This is what you've been waiting for. Let's get to it. He walked to the kitchen, put the dish, fork, and pan in the dishwasher, and returned the condiments to their respective perches. Next he went upstairs. It was slow going—his ears were ringing. Breathing crowded him. With trembling hands, he took an overnight bag out of the hall closet and set it on the bed. He should have had a suitcase packed. His friends, Jerry and Mary, said they had her bag packed weeks before their baby, Tommy, was due. Always best to be ready, they said—just in case. Well, it was too late for "just in case," and he wasn't giving birth to a new life. Instead, he was getting one—a fine, healthy new kidney.

"This has to be right. This just has to be right," he told himself.

He stared at the overnight bag on the bed. What would he need? Toothbrush, electric shaver, what else? Yes, a long robe to cover those damned hospital gowns. The small bag was nearly filled. He threw in a paperback that he had been reading, dropped in his slippers, and zippered the three sides shut.

Then he sat on the edge of the bed, thinking about Martha again. Should he call her now? He vacillated back and forth. She'd be very angry with him for holding back on her. Maybe he'd better wait until he had something definite from the hospital. This could be a false alarm. Only today, Mimi, the nurse in the clinic, had warned him.

"Now when you do get the call, remember it's not certain," she had said. "We could have an antigen problem, or something could undermine the kidney before it's removed or delivered here. You'll be all excited when the call comes, but stay realistic. Things can go wrong."

Well, nothing was going to go wrong with his new kidney!

He put his billfold in his pocket, removed it and checked for their phone credit card. It was there. He added the piece of paper with the phone number of Martha's hotel. She always left her itineraries and appropriate phone numbers whenever she had to be gone over night.

He walked down the steps, scarcely knowing what he was doing, moving on automatic pilot. He got his jacket and a cap from the closet, sat down, checked the directory for the cab company phone number, then placed the call. Just as he hung up, he remembered the answering machine. Erasing the tape, he programmed a new outgoing message:

"Thanks for calling. Please leave a message at the beep." He was about to stop there, but he knew that wasn't enough. "Martha, check the hospital."

He walked to the kitchen and looked around. Satisfied that he'd cleaned up the dishes and food after himself, he returned to the front room and stood silently, trying to calm his rising excitement. He heard the cab's horn as it pulled up to the house.

Yes, he told himself, it's time to go. Bag in hand, he opened the front door and walked outside.

27

CRANKING UP

4:00 A.M.

"The numbers will be worn off that damned clock from all this staring at it. Why don't we hear something?" Carolyn drummed her fingers on the desk. "I hate uncertain waiting."

Max was already pacing the floor, getting up steam—ready to take the liver to the airport and a kidney to Memorial Central. It would be hours before he was needed for those runs, but he was chomping at the bit to get the process started.

"You must have been a Boy Scout," she said to him.

He paused and looked confused.

"You know—'always prepared,'" she added.

Suddenly, her pager went off and everyone around her jumped. She grabbed a phone and called the switchboard.

"Carolyn, we just got a patch from the highway patrol. They're out of Hinkley. Roads and visibility clearing. Should be here in an hour and a half."

"Thanks, Jean. We've been waiting for that." She hung up the phone. "All right, everybody. Our man on the road will be here in an hour and a half."

Max strode to the large, numeric timer.

"Eighty minutes and counting," he said, wisely setting it on the short side.

Carolyn looked over at him. "That should give us plenty of time to be ready when they get here. Is the weather holding to the south?"

He nodded. She picked up her clip board, scanned it, and turned to face the others around her, a mingling of call nurses and general staff still on duty from the donor's original surgery.

"All right, we need to crank up our readiness here. Max, call Meg at Rochester Mercy. She's already standing by. Give her the e.t.a. on Mr. Popovich, and tell her we'll keep her informed as we get into gear." Max smiled. He knew she hated promising schedules that could fall apart at any time.

"Max, make sure who's to order the charter. If she's not yet tied into some line there, recommend our guys. That would be easier on this end. But she's being pushed a lot tonight, and this her first time alone. So feel it out, and do what she wants." In addition to his other qualities, Max was a tactful diplomat. She turned back to the assembly.

"Marian, talk to Becky. She may need help setting up for Hartung. They'll be back in One for harvest. Dolan will go to Two for the transplant." Marian nodded.

"Patsy, check that stereo in One. Someone said it quit during the earlier surgery. If it's not working, ask Max to look at it when he's free. He's good at jiggling wires. Maybe John Philip Sousa will keep Hartung awake during that removal. He's already had a long night." Everyone within earshot laughed. Hartung's propensity for catching sleep at odd moments due to his hectic schedule was well-known.

Patsy moved out of the circle with a nod of assurance.

"Jimmy, gather all time data and give Memorial Central the word. Their recipient is on the way in and doing well, but

Mimi needs to be kept up-to-date. She told us to go ahead with their harvest. Her implant surgeon is on his way in—from halfway across the continent, to hear Mimi tell it.

"Dr. Sciaretta will transplant one kidney here this morning. I've reserved Three for him. I suspect he'll do the removal. Might be good to page Nancy Martinez to be certain. Then make notes on my board and also inform Dr. Hartung. We'll let him decide who's to do Memorial Central's kidney excisions, and when to call any extras he needs. Just keep everyone informed."

Spotting Max out of the corner of her eye, she added.

"Max, I've volunteered your electronic genius to Patsy in One. Then, coordinate with Jimmy on the transportation to Memorial Central. You can just hail down a courier when their kidney is ready."

"I starts 'em, I finishes 'em," he replied, a quirky grin on his face.

"Whatever you say." Carolyn enjoyed the loyal camaraderie of this bunch.

She turned her attention back to the undulating circle milling about the nurses' station.

"Georgie, Nancy Martinez is meeting Sciaretta over at Greenwood to check the patient. They should be back here with Mrs. Lonsdale in about an hour. Arrange to meet them here. Find a room for the patient, and plan to stay with her while Nancy finishes the transfer papers. See what you can do to prep the patient—begin immunos, or whatever Nancy needs you to do." Georgie snapped her fingers, turned, and left the group.

She looked at Karen, one of the other nurses, who waited expectantly for her assignment.

"I haven't seen Betty yet tonight." Carolyn said. The Heart Boss's chief nurse certainly should be here by now, but, since she never found it necessary to notify Carolyn when she arrived, it always left a blank on Carolyn's chart.

"She's *calling forth* Dr. Dolan's nursing team in one of

the conference rooms for their prerequisite pep talk." Karen made the report with a sly grin. Heart people had the reputation for believing they were ordained to the highest calling. That legend was fairly wide-spread. But of course, Carolyn never believed such rumors—well, hardly ever. Nevertheless, we have to handle them with kid gloves, she thought. There's a definite pecking order.

"Better inform her of our schedule. Make sure the Heart Boss is on his way in. They'll be starting up in OR-One before long." Though protocol indicated that the procurement coordinator called the heart surgeon before making any decisions, his head nurse is generally given the honor of the final call to the surgeon. Carolyn hoped Betty had already signaled that call.

"And tell her Macrae is with the alternate somewhere. I don't know where yet." She thought for an instant. "Will you follow up on that also, Karen, and inform Betty?" Karen nodded, then disappeared.

Again Carolyn checked her clip board and looked up. The circle had shrunk.

"Barbara, want to get your feet wet?" Barbara's smiling expression answered her question. New on the job in Emergency Room surgery, but carrying excellent surgical credentials, she'd indicated an interest in transplant work. Might as well give her a start tonight.

"Hang on a minute." Carolyn turned. "Ruth, may I assume our donor is holding?"

"Indeed." she replied. "The aunt's friend has been with him most of the time."

"In about ten minutes you'd better give them a two-minute warning, then bring him back. We need him prepped and ready in One before the Hartung convocation."

Staff hustled in and out, fulfilling their assignments. Carolyn issued a broad message.

"All right, everyone. You have maybe an hour for R and R."

A few snickers acknowledged that they understood her exaggeration.

"I want someone covering this phone from now until the morning shift comes in. And the last person on is to brief the replacement. I want four people on stand-by to meet the ambulance and get the patient into the building, onto one of our carts, and ready for surgical prep without a second's delay. We'll need two nurses for starting and/or replacing drips. We'll probably need to clean him up a bit before moving him into the OR to be prepped. All this should flow in one, smooth wave that will deliver Mr. Popovich to Betty in Two. Settle on your jobs with one another. Do whatever needs doing." She thought for an instant. "Oh, yes, take breaks as needed, in rotation, well ahead of the deadline."

For a moment chaos reigned as everyone ran into one another, then order quickly took over as they settled into their roles. Almost immediately, they looked like a team again.

"Now, Barbara, I'm giving you these sheets. Everything is on them. We'll have two organs to go." She waited for Barbara's reaction, and got a smile. "And two staying here. The Heart Boss—if you haven't guessed—is Dr. Dolan. Dr. Mike Sciaretta is noteworthy for kidneys. Both are regulars here."

"I've worked with Dolan on open heart cases."

"Good. Then you understand about our little nickname here for him."

"Not just here," Barbara said. They both chuckled.

"Well, for tonight I'd like you to play traffic cop at this station until the two organs are gone and the other two are delivered to their respective ORs. Just check off everything on these lists as it is completed." Barbara nodded continuously. "But don't ever guess. If you don't know what's happening, ask the person involved, or—better still—ask me."

Carolyn scanned the area. The circle had evaporated. They all knew their jobs, and now it was time to get ready for

action. She handed Barbara the sheets, listing standard procedures, names of assigned people, and her scribbled notes down
one side.

"Run a copy of these, will you, Barbara? I'll want a set for
my final reports." And to keep count with you, she thought to
herself. Nothing was to be left to chance, especially with a rookie.

Barbara ran through the checklist, then nodded to
Carolyn, who spoke again.

You'll notice that we kid around a lot within the teams. We
do it to keep from losing our minds over the tragedy we face at
every cadaver transplantation. But our recipients are ill. So, when
they are within hearing range, we moderate our voices, or skip
the jokes altogether. They don't know our bantering is our lifeline. To them, it may well sound callous. This night means only
one thing to each potential recipient and family: a chance for a
future. Soon you will develop an instinct for exactly how close-by
each patient is and when and where laughter is appropriate."
Barbara returned a smile.

"Enough said. Now get to work."

"Aye aye, sir—or is it madam?" The words were spoken
quietly, with only the slightest trace of mockery.

"A simple okay' will do." This one is a fast learner,
Carolyn thought. That was a good sign.

4:15 A.M.

The ambulance carrying Rudy Popovich picked up speed
as the weather cleared. They stopped at Hinkley and the two men
up front got out of the vehicle. From what she could hear, Jan
knew that the trucks and plows would leave them now, but the
Highway Patrol was staying on—just in case they ran into problems ahead.

She wanted to go out and thank all those who had helped
them make this treacherous trip through the blizzard, but she

didn't want to let the cold into the back of the ambulance. Besides, this was only a portion of the many people involved. She would find a way to thank them in letters, later, when she and Rudy got home again. Those words sounded strange now. She wondered when that would be.

They were on the move again. The worst was over, thank God. Jan settled back onto her hard perch, steadied by the corner walls of the cabin. She tried to stay awake but, exhausted, soon nodded off to sleep.

Suddenly, she sensed something was wrong. As she snapped open her eyes, she saw trouble etched on Julie's face. Jan looked at her husband. Rudy was struggling for breath and thrashing his arms in panic. Julie tried to get the ventilator mask onto his face. Suddenly his arms dropped, useless. Jan wanted to do something, but she was paralyzed with fear.

Quickly, Julie adjusted the ventilator settings. Holding the mask in place with one hand, she tried to open the black bag she had brought. But Rudy's panic revived itself, and again he tried to grab the ventilator tube.

"It's all right, Rudy. I'm just giving you a good blast of oxygen and something to help you feel better." Jan suddenly came to life and slid next to Julie and opened the satchel.

Julie nodded a thank you. "It's Okay, Jan. He'll be all right." She removed a swab from the bag and gave it to Jan to open.

"Pull his sleeve up as far as you can." Jan moved quickly to her knees and held Rudy's bare arm steady while Julie cleaned a patch of skin. Next, Julie took a syringe from the open bag, pulled the protective end off with her teeth, and plunged the needle into Rudy, emptying its contents.

"Try to breathe naturally, Rudy. Just relax. You're doing fine. We haven't far to go anymore." His body seemed to go limp again.

Jan's earlier joy burst in flames of terror as she pushed

herself away. In dread, she watched Rudy's pallid face, and saw his whole body go slack.

Julie leaned forward and pointed at the window of the cab. She put a finger to her lips, pointed again to the window and then to her watch. When the attendant responded, Jan tried to look calm. She mimicked Julie's signals.

The attendant looked at his watch, mouthed some words and held up fingers to indicate forty-five minutes. He seemed to understand that the patient was in trouble.

He pointed to the roof; Julie nodded.

Jan felt dread submerging her. No, no, no, she wanted to shout. Rudy can't die. Not here, not now.

The ambulance emitted one short, shrill blast of siren. Jan looked at her husband. Rudy did not react. The highway patrol car responded with one short blast, then launched into full ahead, with siren blaring, as the ambulance raced to keep up.

Jan shivered. The iciness came from within. She watched Rudy. He was quiet now, frighteningly quiet. Was it the medication Julie administered? She had to believe Julie knew what needed to be done under these circumstances.

Jan squeezed her eyes and fists shut, then pounded the fists on her thighs. You head-strong Croate, why did you waste all that strength trying to be a comedian? The doctor told you to save your energy. Why couldn't you have slept as you were supposed to? Fearful and anxious, her mind raced out of control.

Then, just as suddenly, she drew in the reins. She must be calm. She must stay aware. She must pray. That was the best thing she could do.

She knelt beside the stretcher and stroked Rudy's cold forehead. Again and again she caressed that soft, silver hairline. She would keep him alive with the warmth of her love if that's what it took. He had to live. He had to.

She felt Julie's hands on her shoulders, gently kneading the tight muscles. In the distance, up ahead, she heard the siren on the Patrol car. They were driving terribly fast. With her free hand she grasped the side rail of the stretcher to keep from falling. But she never lost touch of Rudy's brow.

She prayed they would make it.

4:20 A.M.

Father John explained he needed some time to be with Michael. Soon after he left, Margaret dozed off, her rosary twisted around her fingers. The chanting pattern of the recitation had been the soothing tranquilizer she needed.

When she awakened, she looked at the clock. It had been a long time since she had heard anything from the doctors or nurses. Perhaps she should go back to Donald again. Maybe this time she would be stronger, better prepared. She pulled herself to her feet, and shuffled toward the room where Donald's body waited.

Nothing had changed. Her gasp, over which she had no control, startled Michael and Father John.

"I checked on you and thought you were asleep," the priest said. "Did you get a little rest?"

She nodded. "He looks so cold," she said. Choked with tears, she turned away. In silence, she composed herself, pulled herself up to full posture, and turned back toward the table.

"They said it was almost time," Michael said.

"Someone came in to tell you that?"

"Nurses and doctors have been coming in frequently to check the monitors, feel his pulse, and listen to his heart. Most of them haven't said anything. But Carolyn, the young woman from the organ procurement center, was the last one in, and she said they were nearly ready." Margaret nodded.

"She also said they had a critically ill man with nine children coming by ambulance through a blizzard for the transplant of Donny's heart." He paused, fighting tears.

"Imagine that, nine children," she said. "What if he doesn't make it?"

"Carolyn said they have another man ready, just in case. He's here in the hospital."

"I hope the man with the nine children makes it."

Father John pulled a chair next to the wheelchair for Margaret. Michael put his arms around her shoulders. When she calmed, she looked in her purse for some fresh tissues. There were none. She had to dig into her coat pocket for the old, soggy ones. She tried to wipe her face with the sodden mass. Watching her, Father John drew a clean handkerchief from his pocket and gave it to her.

They waited quietly with their separate thoughts, memories. Margaret was too numb now to think about anything. She needed this to be over.

Two nurses came into the room. One busied herself with arranging equipment. The other crouched in front of Margaret and Michael. She spoke softly, reverentially.

"We'll be taking Mr. Mills to the operating room now. I hope it will comfort you to know that your generosity is making possible a priceless gift for four very sick people and their families." Margaret nodded—habit, perhaps. She felt nothing.

The nurse stood again, giving each of the three a direct glance. Her face and tone of voice were kind and caring.

"You should leave now. It has been a very long night for all of you. There's nothing you can do here anymore."

Margaret and Michael huddled together, Father John next to them, each connected by hand to the others, until the nurses drew the curtains and moved Donald and the equipment out of the cubicle. Then, they followed into the semi-darkened corridor and stood silently as Donald's body was moved away from them down the long hallway. The nurses walked slowly until they reached a brighter lit passageway that veered to the left. As they turned, Donald's body was gone.

Margaret spoke—to no one, really.

"His life meant something, didn't it?" It was something that plagued her.

"Of course it did, Mrs. Bond," Michael said in a tear-filled voice. "His life mattered to me. He kept me alive all these years."

She only barely heard Father John's quiet whisper. "May his soul, and all the souls of the faithful departed, rest in peace. Amen."

28

OPENING NIGHT

4:25 A.M.

Carolyn leaned against the nursing station counter to watch the procedure. It was like opening night every time multiple donor transplantations happened. The tension and excitement had built with each of the twenty-plus new arrivals. Crummy hours and middle-of-the-night pilgrimages through thunder storms or below-zero temperatures couldn't defuse their eagerness. Nor the palpable tension of waiting when they finally arrived at the appointed place. Nor tired legs and aching backs during the long sieges over the operating table.

Once they had participated in the planting of new life, they were snared, captivated, addicted to this life-and-death work. To a stranger, seeing them hasten through the doors singly or in clusters of twos and threes, there would be no way to distinguish what role each was to play in this night's drama. Who would be the surgeon? The scrub nurse? The surgical resident ready to study at the side of the master? The casualness of their dress kept their secret.

This morning they hurried in, filled with purpose, tinged with the crispness of the Minnesota night's air. They called out or waved greetings with unbroken motion. Light conversation flowed with their forward moves. They knew where their costumes awaited them—green, unisex, two-piece suits, matching shoe covers to pull over the jogging shoes most of them wore everywhere now. No one needed a mirror to pull on and adjust the generic green which would cover their hair. The final touch: surgical masks tied in place across faces, then dropped to their chests, ready to be returned to position before entering the operating room. Complete uniformness. And yet, as they congregated, waiting for the opening curtain, that bland, identicalness of the costume spotlighted the readiness of each face.

No matter how often she'd witnessed this opening night rite, Carolyn was always awed by the aggregation of this ensemble cast, primed for the night's production. They are awesome, Carolyn thought.

As Tom Hartung arrived at the nurses' station, an inaudible signal summoned everyone to the surrounding area. Hartung picked up his clip board and faced the group.

"Okay, everyone, listen up. In OR One, donor Donald Mills is being prepared."

Carolyn felt the excitement of this moment. The director's briefing to the cast for tonight's performance. Every eye was fixed upon him. A nurse who had been chewing gum stopped instantly with his first word. The august Heart Boss, Dr. Dolan, in full costume, had joined the gathering. Even he stood motionless, listening intently. The small muscles between his jaw and ears flexed ever so slightly. The star of tonight's drama, surely he knew his lines. But he knew also it was crucial that he listen now to the director. To hear every nuance, to sense every mood of other cast members.

"We have no idea," Hartung began, "what our primary heart recipient's condition will be. We have to be prepared for anything."

They were nodding their heads—in affirmation, or simply in comprehension. He had them all. Their attention riveted on him. They were ready. Scene One was about to begin.

4:30 A.M.

Nancy Martinez arrived at the nursing station where Bob Lonsdale had been nervously waiting. As she came into view, he remembered meeting her the day Kate was placed on the waiting list for a donor kidney.

"Good to see you again, Mr. Lonsdale."

"Bob, please." He shook her hand. "I can't tell you how good it is to see you."

"That's what all my recipient families tell me." Her smile was warm and reassuring. "Did you tell Kate about the transplant?"

"No, though I thought about it. I decided to wait for Dr. Ben."

Dr. Ben Osborne soon arrived, exuding good cheer.

"What a wonderful night this is to be," Dr. Ben said. "Thank you for including me."

Dr. Sciaretta's car, he reported, was just entering the parking ramp as he walked to the elevator. "By the way, Robert— please don't think I'm meddling, but what about Kate's parents, the Landers?"

"They'll be here on the first available flight," Bob said. The doctor smiled and nodded approval. Bob was grateful for the man's compassion—and tact.

For the first time since her condition had worsened to the point where death seemed inevitable, Kate radiated when told about the transplant. She asked to see the baby and held Kathleen close, a bright, serene smile on her face. A few minutes later, when the baby had to be taken back to the nursery, Kate was ready. The doctors left with cheerful promises to see her in surgery. Nancy went out with them.

"I have to finish some paper work," she said.

As Kate drifted off to sleep, Bob's mind raced through his mental list. The Landers will be here later this morning. Nurses were canceled for now. ICU will keep Kathleen for a day or two. He would need to settle the Greenwood bill, but he was sure that could wait. His brain bounced from one idea to another. He felt frenzied with excitement as he groped for practicality.

What else am I forgetting? No need to call the office until after the surgery. All his appointments for the day were rescheduled when he planned on taking Kathleen home.

The ambulance crew came into the room, wheeling their stretcher next to the bed.

"We're going now," Bob said, as Kate awakened.

"For my new kidney and our new life," she said with a certainty that amazed Bob. Again she glowed with joy as she and the tubes that were sustaining her were lifted with great care onto the cart.

All the nurses on duty stood outside the station to give Kate their farewells and best wishes. She raised her arm up onto her elbow, and each nurse grazed her hand across Kate's, a team cheering on a scoring teammate.

The tears in Kate's eyes could not dampen her new smile.

Nancy joined the hurried pace toward the elevators.

"Nancy, are we in a rush?" Bob asked.

"Well, we're not on emergency status, though we do need to get going."

Bob pointed down the long hall, toward the baby's neonatal ICU.

"Just five minutes?" He pleaded.

Nancy turned to the attendants.

"If Dr. Sciaretta complains, we blame Mr. Lonsdale. We were hijacked, right?" The men laughed and nodded, a little unsure about the joke. She turned back to Bob,

"Lead on." He took off in a run.

At the entrance to the nursery, where Bob had disappeared, Nancy rolled Kate onto her side. Within seconds Bob returned, gowned, breathless, and carrying a round loaf of blanket and baby.

"Your daughter wants to cheer you on, too, Kate," Bob said as he laid the wiggling bundle down on Kate's arm.

The moment seemed frozen in time. Kate touched the tiny head, the sweet, clear white face, and then the tiny fingers of her baby.

"I love you, Kathleen," she whispered. "I'll be back with you very soon."

4:35 A.M.

The countdown clock showed sixty minutes. Maybe I have time for just one fresh cup of coffee, Carolyn thought. Just then her pager signaled.

"What have you got, Jean?" As she listened, her face sobered. Everyone within range turned to watch her.

"Oh, No!" The group seemed to slump collectively into a stunned silence, all eyes locked on Carolyn.

"It's all right, Jean. This isn't your fault. We'll be ready. Thanks." Carolyn looked up at the worried faces.

"Listen up, everybody. Our heart recipient is in bad shape. They're pulling out all the stops. Should be here in something near thirty minutes, and we've got to be ready to prep and open him STAT—if he's still alive."

Now, everyone moved at double time. Carolyn put out a page for Macrae. No time for finding lost people now.

"Karen, get the word to Betty."

The nurse nodded and rushed out.

Macrae returned her page. "Your primary is now on accelerated approach, sirens screaming." Carolyn explained. "They estimate thirty minutes, but his heart is bad. Better have number two readied."

Two lives seemed to be hanging by a thread.

Carolyn walked to the scrub area and reported the emergency. Dr. Dolan's shoulders dropped. His expression was grim as he turned toward her.

"We'll proceed. I hope the poor devil makes it in time after getting this close."

4:40 A.M.

The telephone dragged Jim and Alicia Goodwin from a deep, relaxed sleep. The first they'd had in a long time. Alicia knew it could only be one of two calls. She said a silent prayer before picking up the phone.

"Mrs. Goodwin?"

"Yes, hello . . ." Alicia's heart pounded furiously.

"This is Meg Tyler from the transplant center. We have good news. We think we have a liver for Patty."

29
ON THE WAY

4:45 A.M.

The best moments of this job, Meg had come to realize, were telling desperately ill patients and their families that the transplants they had been waiting for were finally available.

Alicia Goodwin was too excited to speak after Meg gave her the news. Without a word she handed the phone to her husband. The introverted, usually aloof, man sounded only moments from tears when Meg repeated the good news.

"I don't know how to thank you," he kept repeating. Then, suddenly, he became quiet. Except for the sounds of his breathing, Meg might have thought they'd been disconnected. She was about to ask if he was all right, when he finally spoke.

"I never asked anybody this question. Now I have to know. Just how dangerous is this operation? Could our little girl die during the surgery?"

It was a perfectly rational question, still Meg was taken aback. Why hadn't this come up earlier? It was her fault. She had assumed that the question of risk had been discussed. Perhaps it had been referred to earlier, but didn't register then. Now, however, just when she was giving the Goodwins a message of hope, Meg didn't want them to be frightened.

"Well, Mr. Goodwin, I can't tell you there's no danger. Any surgery has certain risks—even minor ones. But every surgery at this hospital is handled with the utmost care. Dr. Jamison is a highly respected surgeon, and he has performed dozens of liver transplants." Meg did not mention that Patty's would be the first split liver procedure done at Mayo. That was Dr. Jamison's job.

"There's no guarantee. This will be a long, very delicate procedure. But because Patty's illness came on so quickly, the rest of her body has not deteriorated to the point many liver disease patients have. Her present condition is very grave, but she certainly has a high probability of making it through beautifully."

She grasped for something more to say. Quit while you're ahead, woman, she told herself.

"Fair enough," he said somberly. "That's what I needed to know. We'll be there in an hour."

The line went dead. Meg cradled the phone on her shoulder while she let loose a long, slow breath. Congratulations, kiddo. You handled that just about right. Maybe you're going to make it as a coordinator, after all.

She called pharmacy to order medications for Patty, then turned her attention to the charts.

Much of what was in Patty's thick folder was in Meg's own handwriting, beginning with her first day at Mercy Hospital and her initial visit with Dr. Smith. Meg had been called in almost immediately. Dr. Smith knew without any test results how sick Patty was, but an evaluation was required before she could be placed on the national transplant list.

First, however, the hospital's business office had to check on the family's health insurance coverage. Meg hated that part.

Everybody did. Money should not be the first criterion for getting a life-saving organ transplant. But the hospital had no means of supporting the high procurement and implant costs. It wasn't fair, but there was no alternative. Ironically, some years back, kidney transplants for patients of any age, had been placed under the umbrella of Medicare. But none of the other transplants were covered. She had been relieved when Patty's health insurance company approved the surgery.

Page after page recorded the results of days' worth of testing. She read every one again. One was for lung function, and another sheet indicated results of a fine, normal electrocardiogram. An abdominal ultrasound to check blood flow to the liver followed. If the flow had been blocked by disease, a transplant would have been impossible. CAT scan results followed a cancer screening. Even at so young an age, Patty had to be tested for HIV, standard procedure now. All results had been more than satisfactory. Meg had practically memorized the pages, but, each time she read them, she spotted some small item she had not noticed before. She was determined to learn *everything* she would be expected to know about this and all other pre-transplant patients.

The final step had been psychological evaluations of Patty and her parents. The team had to know that Patty, along with her parents, understood and would be committed to doing everything necessary to prevent Patty from abusing her new organ and to help her in the life-long fight against rejection. Meg carefully scrutinized this part. All three had passed this issue with flying colors.

Finally Meg came to the page bearing the formal notation. Diagnosis: fulminant hepatitis. Treatment: transplantation. And Patty had been placed on the national waiting list.

But the rampaging hepatitis had assailed Patty's system with terrifying velocity. And there were no assistance devices to take over for a diseased liver. Her body retained high measures of fluid, and she tumbled into long hours of sleep, slipping perilously close to coma.

Normally, this period of waiting for a donor liver was used to "spiff up" the patients' general health and get them into the best possible shape for their transplant. For Patty's ICU nurses, however, every hour was now intense warfare aimed at keeping her conscious and alive, and preventing brain damage.

The fax machine signaled a new incoming message. One by one the pages of data came in, outlining the test results of Donor 1126.

Forty-six years old—that certainly seemed old for the donation of an organ to a little girl. Same age as Dr. Jamison, Meg recalled. Maybe it wasn't so old after all, she decided. She laid the donor and recipient reports side by side on the nursing station counter. Beginning at the top she worked her way down the pair of files, nodding as she read and checking the top of each page as she matched them. All lab tests had been completed on both patients. Nothing was missing. Patty's x-rays and scans were there in a large separate envelope. She fingered through them, checking each off on her pre-op list. The donor's pictures would accompany his liver. There was nothing she could do about those now.

She placed the charts in two baskets bearing the labels: *Jamison Pre-Op* and *Donor*. Jamison expected the charts to be in the appropriate containers, and always on the exact same spot before each surgery. She gave both packets a snapping pat.

"There!" she uttered. Another job finished.

Phone calls began to come in, inquiries from residents and interns throughout the Mayo staff interested in the split liver surgery. The big news had traveled fast, as Meg had expected. There would be a full house.

Now it was time to begin another list of procedures.

Meg checked her watch. Carolyn's call indicated that Dr. Hartung would soon make the first cut. Since the donor's reports showed no previous surgeries, access would be easier, cutting surgery time to a minimum. She clicked off the time increments, then scheduled a courier for airport pickup of the prized cargo. The plane's e.t.a. was 10:00 A.M.

She called Maureen to check on Patty, and ordered the start of a slow drip of immunosuppressant. Though the OR had already been reserved, she also needed a bed and staff for post-op recovery. She called in the request, then alerted the lab of possible last-minute tests. Lastly, she reserved Patty's bed back in ICU, simply a formality.

"Very good, " she assured herself. "We're ready to go." Timed perfectly with her pronouncement, Dr. Charles Jamison appeared, swooshing both doors open in his wake.

"How goes it, Meghan, my sweet Irish lass?" She felt herself blush. But she refused to be flustered. Remember, you're a professional, she told herself.

"Everything is ready, sir." She hoped it was.

He stood glancing at the two piles of charts. "Look pretty good so far, don't they?"

"Yes, sir." She felt tongue-tied. "They do."

"Any word from the Goodwins?"

"They'll be here," She glanced at her watch again. "Probably within an hour."

"And our liver?"

"I was just working on that. They're close to opening, so it looks to me like it will be a good six-and-a-half hours, counting transportation."

"That long? How much transport time are we looking at?"

"An hour, ground to ground, plus a half hour at each end."

"That's too much time wasted. I want that organ sooner. Order a chopper; that will save us better than an hour. I should have skipped the search for a surgeon in the twin cities; we could have had our team up in time. Well, that's water under the bridge—but remind me next time. Now, see what you can work out for a chopper."

"Will do." Another new twist. Meg was already revising her to-do list. Cancel the courier to the airport, she thought.

"Well, I'd best get up there to see our little Patty. We don't want anything happening to her before we get that liver here." He turned to leave, then stopped to look at his watch.

"Meghan, put in a call to Adrienne, will you?" He looked at his watch. "Make it about seven o'clock. We might as well give her a little extra time to sleep." He smiled, as if reading her mind.

"See, I'm not totally heartless. Next time, I'll try to give *you* additional sleep time." He pushed open the large double doors leading to the main hospital corridor, then turned back again.

"If Hartung calls through the switchboard, page me, please. See you later."

A long breath escaped in a rush. Well, so far so good, Meg thought. She phoned transportation to begin the search for a helicopter.

4:50 A.M.

"Where to, Mister?" the cab driver asked.

"Memorial Central, please."

"That's way over in Minneapolis."

"Sure is." Roger noticed that he was being eyed in the rear view mirror. He wished the driver would keep his eyes on the road.

"Turned out pretty nice tonight," the driver said, watching the mirror for Roger's response. "But I guess tomorrow may be the end of it, and we'll be back to January again."

Roger muttered a reply. A talkative cabbie is all I need tonight, he thought. Then he realized the guy was just being pleasant.

"You have a point there." Roger thought his remark sounded irrelevant, but what do you say to a complete stranger who obviously wants conversation on the night shift? He wished he'd gotten the poet again.

The streets were nearly deserted. As they hit the Highland Village area, the holiday lights were welcoming, though the brightness only heightened the look of desertion. The lamp posts were still wrapped in greens from the holidays. Roger remembered those adornments from his childhood. On Christmas night, en route home from Grandma's, his father would drive through the Village to see the street lights and store decorations. They weren't on the grand scale of the downtown shopping areas, but this was his father's own special tradition. Since there was rarely any other traffic up Ford Parkway, Pop used to say the Village put on this show "just for our little family."

The Village isn't the same anymore, Roger thought—bigger, some parts better, others more impersonal. The big department store was new—"convenient," Martha said. But the papers reported that it was soon to be closed for lack of business. Other shops seemed to come and go too quickly to become a habit. Roger's favorite new haunt, however, was a half-price book shop, cornerstone of a new strip mall. He loved that store, with its smell of old books. That was about all his shopping budget allowed anymore, half-price old books. But Pat, his favorite clerk, always greeted him with a selection of new arrivals she was sure he'd like. And she was always right on the money.

Funny, Roger thought, until just now he had forgotten those annual Christmas night drives through the Village. What else had he forgotten about his father? He smiled, remembering some very special times from his childhood.

They were crossing the Ford Bridge into Minneapolis.

"Driver, will you take the loop to the right, down to the river, before we go to the hospital?"

"It's your dollar, Mister. We can go anywhere you want." The driver made a right turn at the next intersection. Roger was aware that the man was studying him more seriously in the mirror and turned his face toward the side window, trying to shut out anything outside his own thoughts.

"Any place in particular you want to see?" the driver asked as he turned onto River Drive.

"Stop in the next block, will you?"

"Like I say, it's your dollar." The driver pulled to the curb, giving Roger a full look into the darkness that hung over the river. Snow banks along the road obscured his view of the river itself.

Roger stared out the window, then opened the cab door.

"I'll just be a few minutes, if you don't mind."

"Just so you know, the meter keeps running." Roger heard the distrust in the driver's voice.

"Don't worry, I won't be long. You'll get your money."

He slammed the door a bit too sharply. But what did it matter? He would tip the driver well for this trip.

He climbed the snow bank, and walked to the bank ledge, looking down the six-foot embankment to the shoreline. Scattered lights glistened off the ice and snow spread across the Mississippi. He walked a half-block or better to the north. Yes, this was the spot.

After Roger had recovered from rheumatic fever, his dad took him fishing several times, right along this area. He taught Roger to bait a hook, to cast his line, and to play a fish until he could bring it to shore. Roger hadn't been too keen on reaching into the muddy can of worms and threading the slippery creatures onto the hook—nor removing a fish from the hook. But he loved the time alone with his dad.

"Some day, Rogie," the old man would say, "we'll get us a

boat. And then we can go fishing anywhere we want. Why we can follow the river all the way down to New Orleans and into the Gulf of Mexico, where the really big ones will be waiting for us."

But a street cop's pay was never enough to buy a boat. And when the promotions came, there wasn't time anymore to go fishing or boating. Later, Roger understood. When his father was dying, Roger was just beginning his first job. Then it was his turn to make the promise that couldn't be kept. "You get well, Pop, and we'll get that boat and go fishing all the way down to New Orleans." His father smiled. Roger was sure they each had meant the promise when it was made. "I'm sorry, Pop." His silent words crept across the years of lost dreams. "I wish we could have done it together."

Roger heard the footsteps crackle off the crisp, wet grass. For an instant he stiffened in fear. Then he made out the silhouette of the cab driver's flapping ear protectors.

"You all right, fella?" the man asked.

"Yes. We can go on now."

Back in the warm vehicle the air seemed stuffy. Roger rolled down the window a bit, and again he noticed the driver studying him in the mirror.

"You got someone sick in the hospital?" he asked.

"No, I'm the sick one."

"You don't look sick, man."

Roger smiled. "Thanks."

"What kind of sick are you?"

"I'm getting a new kidney tonight, a transplant."

"You don't mean it?" The driver's voice carried a mixture of disbelief and distrust. "How're you gonna' get that?"

"Oh, I guess they have a warehouse of spare kidneys some place."

"We'll, I'll be. This is sure a first for me."

"For me, too," Roger said.

With that, the driver accelerated to breakneck speed.

Roger grabbed hold of the neck rest of the front seat.

"If it's all the same to you," Roger finally managed to say. "I'd really wish to get there in one piece."

The cab never slowed until it came to a sliding stop at the emergency entrance of the hospital. For the moment, at least, Roger's wish had come true.

30

ACT I, SCENE II

4:50 A.M.

The two surgeons stood at the scrub sinks. Hartung had forced himself to shrug off thoughts of the incoming patient. It helped that he did not know the man. Someone would get this heart, regardless. But, as he watched Jonah Dolan stare into space, he saw the face of a doctor deeply moved by the possible loss of the patient.

There were those who scorned Dolan's flair for the dramatic, and his sometimes arrogant facade, but Hartung had known him too long to be put off by such mannerisms. They had been in the same class in medical school at New York University, and then entered surgical residencies together in Iowa. But, while Hartung continued at Iowa, Dolan spent two grueling years in Houston. It was said in medical circles that if you survived Houston, you were invincible; you could save the world. Not only did Jonah survive, he reportedly loved those two years. And Hartung had no doubt that Jonah could, indeed, save the world if he could fit it into his schedule. If Hartung's heart ever gave out, Jonah was the surgeon he would want working on him.

Unfortunately, although they both ended up at Met Gen, their personal lives had taken different directions, especially during Jonah's several divorces and remarriages. Now when their paths crossed at social events—or, as tonight, working on the same cadaver—conversation took on the usual timbre of male intimacy: Super Bowl teams, the poor showing of the Minnesota Timberwolves, and of course, hockey. Tonight was no different as the weather got its share of accolades. But Hartung had seen, however briefly, that gentle side of Jonah he remembered from their early days. Hartung was glad it still remained in the heart of this man who had once been his friend.

Finally they were ready for the patient's arrival and their respective jobs in OR One.

The murmured whispers hushed as Hartung and Jonah Dolan came through the door into the OR, their gloved, sterile hands held high, ready to commence. Hartung stepped up to the table, while Jonah stood aside. The torso of Donald Mills lay in wait, freshly shaved and painted that bright, uneven orange that startles most patients at first sight after surgery. This patient would never know.

His head and loins were covered; the latter with a set of folded sheets that angled up over his hips, and onto the table. The surgical field was fully exposed.

Becky handed the first scalpel to Hartung. He positioned it firmly in his grip, took one deep breath and began. At the top of the sternum, the breast bone, he set the blade and moved with absolute precision down the length of the torso. Then with a small electric saw he split the rib cage. The senior resident, who stood across the table from Hartung, set the clamps on each side of the slightly separated rib cage. With care he turned the handles, triggering the slow spreading of the chest cavity.

His colleague leaned down, searching for a first sight of the heart, even before it was exposed. Hartung's attention was focused on the area of the liver he would be removing. As the wedge gaped wider and the organs came into view, both uttered in unison, "Beautiful." Everyone in the room released long-held breaths.

Dr. Emily McCabe, who had been standing behind the resident, quietly clapped her hands over her head. Carolyn and Macrae watched from near the door. Hartung looked over to them and nodded with satisfaction.

"We got us four beauties here, folks. The music's gonna play tonight." The observers turned and left the room, patting each other on the back.

Dr. Jonah Dolan moved into position. Ever the master showman, he stretched his arms like a professional conductor, paused for attention before signaling for the stereo to begin. He brought down his hands with the first explosion of music.

Hartung reeled slightly from the blast of sound. Go to it, tiger, he said to himself.

4:55 A.M.

One of Rochester's helicopters was out for repairs. Another was on a LifeLine flight, and the third was restricted to local emergencies. So much for the hometown gang, Macrae thought. She reached for the phone once more.

"Carolyn, this is Meg, again. Our little recipient is on shaky ground. Dr. Jamison doesn't want to wait out all that travel time. Do you have a helicopter available?"

"You beat me to the call," Carolyn responded. "We have an emergency of our own coming down—the heart recipient. The surgery has just begun. Hartung should have the job wrapped up in at most four hours. I was in OR for the opening, and everyone is very excited about the excellent condition of our donor organs."

"Sounds great. And the chopper?"

"No problem. I'll put Max on it, and he'll keep you posted. Still your tab?"

"Well, of course." Meg broke into a raucous laugh, which felt very good.

"Don't worry," Carolyn said, "it won't take more than two or three years salary to pay it off.

"We'll keep you informed."

31

VIRTUOSO PERFORMANCE

5:00 A.M.

Tom Hartung stood back for a time, watching Jonah Dolan feel and study the pumping heart. He'd heard Dolan's nickname—the Heart Boss—and he knew it wasn't always meant to be a flattering label—though Jonah, who was aware of it, seemed to accept the term as his proper laurel. That was typical of heart surgeons, Tom had observed. Most he'd met seemed to move about encapsuled within a crystal shell, an aura of imperviousness surrounding them.

It had been several years since Hartung had watched Jonah execute his wizardry. He remembered that last occasion vividly. Hartung had once joined Jonah at the table for a quadruple by-pass. And it was a sight to behold. Like a violinist, Jonah maneuvered his fingers with smooth, swift accuracy.

The patient was Hartung's cousin James, who had wanted Hartung to do the surgery—foolishly believing his big cousin, the surgeon, could fix anything in the human body. But cardiac surgery was not Hartung's arena. Nor would he have wanted to carry the responsibility for his cousin's life. That was something no surgeon would chance.

So, partly to ease his cousin's jitters and partly to see for himself the condition of James's heart, Hartung had assisted at the surgery. Jonah, of course, needed no assistance from anyone to harvest the long vein from James's thigh, and then thread four cuttings, one by one, through that damaged heart.

Today, James remained a picture of health. A tribute to a superb surgeon, Hartung thought. There's not a single anesthesiologist who has a bad word to say about Dolan's skills, even in the most difficult cases. And that, Hartung believed, was the conclusive gauge of a surgeon's competence. He was trying to keep his own slate that clean.

Hartung watched Jonah continue to survey the pulsing heart. For the moment, he had the luxury of time, as everyone waited for Mr. Popovich's arrival. Harvesting of the heart was actually quite simple, compared to transplantation or by-pass. This heart, however, needed special attention to detail. If the primary recipient was sufficiently stabilized to undergo transplantation, this organ would be positioned next to the fellow's own heart, and the donor organ would actually function through the native heart. If the stand-by, Mr. Nichols, became the recipient, it would be a straight-forward replacement. Jonah was obviously thinking of both scenarios as he poised to begin.

Word spread through the OR that the heart patient's ambulance had just crossed the city limits, and that the patient was, for the moment, holding his own. Jonah clenched his hand into a fist, and jolted it with obvious pleasure. Above surgical masks, everyone's eyes showed relief that Rudy Popovich was still hanging on.

From the sidelines, Hartung's attention drifted to the liver. It certainly looked fine from this vantage point. He slipped away unnoticed—back to his office where no one would distract him. The ventilating system gave him a sudden chill as he removed the sweat-saturated cap and mask, then the scrubs. The OR had become miserably warm, an environment critical to maintaining the cadaver stability—more specifically, of the donor liver. Once the removal began, the temperature could be gradually lowered.

Hartung pulled a spare set of underwear and a fresh scrub suit from the storage cabinet. Their dryness felt good, especially when he added a lab coat. He eased his aching back with a few upper body twists and arm reaches, then sat down at his desk. A note rested alone at the center of his desk blotter. Dr. Charles Jamison answered on the first ring.

Jamison soon made it obvious that he did not like "outsiders" harvesting for him. His wish-list of information about the donor liver was actually quite elementary. Perhaps Jamison thought he was the only transplant surgeon in the world who needed measurements—and as much connective tissue as could possibly be gleaned from the donor. Perhaps fatigue caused Hartung's negative reaction, but he also had an MD after his name, and he'd been involved in this harvesting game for nearly a decade.

At any rate, Hartung already had relatively close measurements, just from eyeballing the organ. That, Jamison assured him, was imminently helpful. Of course venous measurements for the undersides would not be available until the organ was free. As they talked, however, Hartung more fully appreciated Jamison's concerns. This donor's arteries would be measurably larger than the recipient's, making attachment more complex—and actually impossible if sufficient tissue was not available. Score one for the Mayo Man.

Hartung promised to have Carolyn send frequent progress reports—and sizes—throughout the surgery.

Hartung returned to the OR just as Jonah severed and

clamped the aorta, the final disconnection of Donald Mills's heart. Slowly, Jonah lifted the now motionless organ from the cadaver's chest. As with every Dolan move in the surgical suite, this, too, seemed ceremonial. Like a high priest presenting sacrifice to the gods, he elevated the organ well above the cavity. It seemed suspended in space, a ritualistic offering, as Jonah studied the surface, the curvature, and each vein stem.

Surely the gods must be pleased, Hartung thought. This was a fine offering.

The heart was then placed into a stainless steel container, filled with a chilled electrolyte solution that would flush and clean the organ, removing all traces of the donor's blood.

Jonah and Hartung spoke briefly as the heart surgeon turned to leave—as always, exuding his confident gait.

Now Hartung had work of his own to prepare for—harvesting a liver for none other than the Mayo Clinic. He turned to the senior resident.

"Probe and lift the area surrounding the liver."

It looked good. Very, very good.

Time to re-scrub. Hartung left the operating room—with no "style" whatsoever, he suspected.

His people, who had been resting during the cardiac detachment, would come in immediately. The newer resident would "tidy up the body." Becky would position her tray of fresh, sterile instruments, and housekeeping would remove trash and replace the container lining before work began on the donor liver. It all went quickly.

Now it was Hartung's turn to play genius.

5:05 A.M.

They were in familiar territory now and Margaret felt a sense of relief. The night had been like a trip to another world, an ugly world of pain and noise —the chaos of the hospital emergency waiting room, seeing Donald in that blank, sterile room. Seeing Donald? Could this have all been a terrible night-mare?

Father John pulled to a stop in front of her house. It's whiteness seemed luminous against the dark sky. It seemed to stare at her, hovering menacingly over the dark area surrounding it. This had been her home for all these years. Inside it, she had always felt warm, safe. But not tonight. She looked up at the dark second floor. There had always been light shining out from those windows when she returned from an evening of cards or a dinner with friends. But not tonight. Part of the house seemed to have died.

She was startled when Father John opened the door beside her. She had forgotten she was still in his car. She felt foolish sit-ting there like a lump. Instinctively, she grasped at her purse clasp. Always have your keys in hand before approaching your home or car, she remembered—a caution from a police officer who spoke to her senior's group. It had become habit, but now her purse refused to open as she fumbled with the buckle. She felt hopelessly flustered.

"It's all right, Margaret. Take your time." Father John said.

Finally, the bag opened and she shuffled through its con-tents until she found the familiar plastic fob. Donald had given it to her. He'd gotten it for a new bank account he had opened. She liked it because it was large and easy to find in her purse. Now, she simply stared at it. She had nearly worn off the gold print-ing. She continued staring at it as she closed her purse. It was such a nice key chain. And Donald had given it to her.

She had lost her sense of time and place until she finally looked up again. She didn't seem to know what to do next. Her brain was scrambled.

"Let me give you a hand, Margaret," Father John said. He reached a hand into the car and grasped her arm. She allowed him to help her out of the car, then steadied herself on the street surface before attempting the curb. He still held her arm.

"Thank you so much." It seemed the only appropriate thing to say.

He helped her as she crossed the small patch of grass, until she got her footing on the smooth city sidewalk.

"I'll be fine now, Father," she said. "There's no need to walk me to the door." Heaven knows she had put him through enough tonight. He should go home and get a bit of sleep before his day started again.

"Let me help you up the steps—at least."

"Thank you, again, but I'm all right." She put all the firmness she could manage into her voice, and he released her arm.

Proud, deliberate footsteps carried her across the sidewalk. With great relief she finally grabbed for the railing beside the first tier of steps. Feeling enormous relief, she clung to the wrought iron stanchion. Donald had installed the railing just last summer. He said he didn't want to look out the window some day and see her sprawled on the sidewalk. She knew what he meant. Donald could never let you know he was just being nice about something.

The tears came from nowhere again. There, in the dark, she lost control and found herself doubled over with anguish.

"Here, let me help you." The voice startled her, terrifying her for just an instant until she realized that Father John was still there. He took her right hand in his, and his strong arm wrapped around her waist. Like an obedient child, she lifted one foot and then the next. Four steps, and then a stretch of straight walkway, and, finally, the last four steps to the door. There had always been a railing on both sides of these stairs.

At the top landing, Margaret stepped back while the priest opened the storm door. Her fingers felt numb as she fumbled with the lock. Father John finally took the key, inserted it easily and pushed the door open for her. One more step and she was over the threshold.

Father John moved beside her into the living room, fumbling for a light.

"The switch is just a few inches from the door on the left."

The room was suddenly filled with light that radiated warmth. It was familiar and protective.

"Is there anyone you would like me to call, Margaret?"

She shook her head. She couldn't think of anyone. All she needed now was to be alone.

"I don't like leaving you here without anyone to be with you."

"I'll be fine, Father," she said. "I just need some rest." Oh, please, she did need to rest!

"Very well, then—if you promise to call me as soon as you wake up." How very kind he was, she thought, and nodded her head slowly. She remained in the hallway to see him out.

Opening the door as he was departing, he spoke again.

"Be sure to lock this, Margaret." Then, just before closing it, he turned again.

"I'm awfully sorry, Margaret. So very sorry. But you have friends, and everything will work out, I promise you."

And then he was gone. The front door was finally closed and she obediently locked it. She looked back at the door to Donald's apartment. No sounds from his television. So very quiet.

Too quiet.

5:20 A.M.

Jim Nichols, the alternate heart recipient, was safely waiting in a holding room near the surgical wing with his wife, Rita. Their stares had followed Macrae's every move. She tried not to focus on the frightened, yet hopeful, expressions they wore. But it was hard to ignore them. As she had arranged Jim's medical equipment and endeavored to make them both comfortable in the barren room, she tried to fill the void with light conversation, hoping to distract them. But it hadn't really worked. Too much was at stake for these people tonight. After taking Jim's vital signs again, she gave them all the reassurances she could muster, then left in search of news.

A pair of nurses stood waiting in the corridor. They were leaning against an empty gurney, ready for Rudy Popovich—or Jim Nichols. As soon as Popovich arrived in the unit, these two would take his vitals, make one last draw of blood, and begin drips of immunosuppressants. They were, indeed, prepared.

Carolyn was on the phone at the nursing station. Macrae waited until she hung up the receiver.

"Any news?"

"Popovich is holding steady," Carolyn reported. "Pulse weak, but stabilized again. Dolan's set-up is completed in Number Two. Your alternate is ready?"

"Ready and hopeful," Macrae said, "though I tried very hard to stress the *if* word. Can you send someone in to wait with them? They're pretty nervous."

Carolyn immediately signaled a passing nurse, and Macrae instructed her. As the young woman moved away, Macrae called after her.

"Please discourage Mrs. Nichols from wandering in this direction. I don't want her spooked." Again the nurse nodded and smiled, then hurried off to her new patient.

"Nancy Martinez called," Carolyn said, "and her kidney patient looks good. They're probably en route. Teresa is overseeing the set up of OR Three for Sciaretta to do the kidney. The other one goes to Memorial Central. Unfortunately, we don't have permission for a tissue take on this one. His aunt was already overwhelmed without explaining the need for tissue transplants."

"And the liver?"

"Ah, that's a rush job—to Rochester. An eight-year-old girl is the recipient. Hartung's excising"

"How do you hang onto all of this?" Macrae asked. "I think I'm being squeezed from both ends with only two people?"

"Remember, I don't get emotionally tied into any of these patients. I'm like the department store Santa. I just dole out the goodies to people I don't even know."

"Never thought of it that way," Macrae said.

"You'll be telling the Nicholses yourself if he has to go back upstairs again?"

"Yes—and you're right about getting emotionally involved. Some, like Jim Nichols, have been here so long, they become like family. And then I've been in regular phone contact with Jan Popovich, especially since this insurance countdown business. It's tough. I just hope we get another heart soon for Jim—if he doesn't get the call tonight."

Macrae felt helplessness wash over her. But she couldn't afford that emotion tonight. Thank goodness this was not her decision to make.

"Thanks, Carolyn," she said as she turned away.

Macrae walked out the ambulance entrance to join several nurses and orderlies who were catching whiffs of the fresh winter evening, trying to revive themselves. Within minutes there was suddenly abrupt silence around her. She caught the distant sound of a siren, screaming louder and closer every second. But so many ambulances come to the hospitals clustered in this part of the city.

"Please, let it be our guy."

Finally she saw the red, flashing lights, then the turn signals—an ambulance lead by highway patrol car, which cut its siren as it turned into the hospital.

"They're here," someone said and ran back inside to sound the call.

The others moved out into position along the driveway. Macrae waited. They knew what had to be done, and how to do it as efficiently as possible. Still, she was nervous. She couldn't help feeling the electric tension in the air.

She focused on the young, red-haired woman running beside the litter, holding up a drip bag and steadying a portable oxygen tank placed next to the patient. An ER nurse positioned herself to match the young woman's pace, took the bag and slapped her hand soundly on the tank. It took several steps for the younger woman to break out of the pattern. Only then did she look up, see the question on Macrae's face, and give a tentative thumbs up.

Macrae walked toward the ambulance where she found Jan Popovich, obviously dazed, making her way out with the help of the driver. She fell into Macrae's arms and sobbed, then struggled to pull herself together as Macrae guided her toward the automatic doors.

"Oh, Macrae, I was so scared. Is he going to make it?"

Before Macrae could respond with an answer she couldn't be sure was true, the young, red-haired woman came over to them and patted Jan's cheek.

"He's all right, Jan, weak but hanging on. He won't quit on us now after we got him this close."

She looked at Macrae. "Hi, I'm Julie. I've been one of Rudy's nurses. I just happened to be off tonight."

Jan was regaining her composure.

"And she insisted on coming along. Rudy would never have made it without her," Jan said. Julie blushed.

Macrae remembered the look. How good to see a nurse go the extra mile. It was surprising how many of them did. At what point do some become a little tired, a little jaded? She wondered.

A wan look on her face, Jan stood watching the ambulance —with Julie—drive out of sight. Macrae understood. The umbilical chord of a secure bond had been cut, now Jan had to face what was ahead alone. Macrae patted her shoulder.

"Don't worry, Jan. Rudy's in very good hands."

About this, Macrae was certain. She just hoped they had gotten the patient here in time.

32

THE O.R./THE WAITING ROOM

5:40 A.M.

Macrae felt guilty having to leave Jan in the waiting room. The poor woman was too bewildered to complain or ask questions. Macrae promised herself that she would get back to her as soon as she could. Right now her patient was the only person that mattered, and she was sure Jan would agree.

A swarm of uniforms was clustered around Rudy's cart, untangling his tubes while removing his hospital gown, preparing his arm for a new IV, then starting new drips, all while flooding him with oxygen. His eyes darted about, then focused on Macrae's face. He began to thrash his arms, trying to speak. Macrae moved closer to the cart.

"Welcome back, stranger."

Tears welled in his eyes and trickled toward his ears in two streams. Once again he tried to speak. Macrae freed the bottom of his ventilator mask.

"It's so good to be here. I never dreamed . . ."

"Save your strength," she said. "We can get caught up

after your surgery. I just want you to know this whole hospital has been cheering you on. And we'll have a real celebration when it's over."

"Is Jan all right?"

"You bet she is." Her conscience niggled. "She's out in the waiting room, and I'll be talking with her regularly during your surgery. So, don't you worry about a thing. Just settle back and enjoy your little nap. I think after this trip you could use one."

He opened his eyes wide to show his awe and happiness, and then closed them.

She ran her hand across his forehead. He felt cold and clammy. Who wouldn't, after such a frightening expedition? She leaned over and whispered, in a very conspiratorial tone.

"You behave yourself, now, and don't give our Heart Boss any trouble. He gets really cranky when patients try to tell him how to do his job."

Rudy's slack jaw firmed and he brought his lips together in one last smile before being slid onto a clean cart and wheeled off into the OR. A cluster of nurses and residents hurriedly began scrubbing, shaving, and painting his upper torso a mustard color. The anesthesiologist stood by, ready to begin intubation of all the additional lines that would be needed during surgery. It's good that only the staff witnesses this scene, Macrae thought. The less a family saw of the frightening aspects of pre-op the better.

But now Macrae would have to talk to the Nicholses. She bit her lip. Why must there always be losers, also-rans?

She decided to hold off on that painful task until the donor heart and the recipient were beyond the point of no return, so to speak. Meanwhile, she walked out to the waiting room to see Jan Popovich.

5:45 A.M.

With fresh clothes and another scrub, Hartung began the liver resection. This time he'd scheduled some Brahms. Finally, he was in position to fully see and feel the organ he had been admiring over the past hour. He was pleased that his preliminary assessment had been correct. This liver was in excellent condition—fine texture, splendid color.

He bent toward it; the liver was the most technically difficult organ for surgical removal. However, the transplantation was a far more arduous procedure, which could take twelve hours, or more, just to implant and reconnect. Hartung's patient had no scars or adhesions from previous surgeries, and he'd already been able to observe the organ during opening. So, he had reason to hope he could accomplish his job in under three hours.

It was obvious, he thought as he called for his first instrument, that Carolyn had taken good care of this donor during the waiting stage, when it was necessary to keep the corpse stable until all assignments were completed for the various surgeries. The liver was the most fragile organ. In addition to a warm environment, it required a careful balance of medical protocols to maintain its healthy condition in a brain-dead patient. The brain monitors and regulates both heartbeat and blood pressure. With the brain no longer sending signals to the heart, the donor can easily become unstable, necessitating medications to sustain blood pressure. And these medications can be toxic to the liver. But there was no problem of toxicity with this liver. Once again the surgeon was impressed by the coordinator's expertise at the handling of donor patients.

The surgery went smoothly without a glitch—and in just over two hours he was finished. Not bad. He knew Carolyn would be relieved. And he was especially pleased that the Mayo people would find no fault with his work or with the liver itself. He turned to watch his staff chill and flush the organ in Wisconsin solution, the standard preparation for all organs now. He wondered how the brew got the Wisconsin label. Probably the developer's ethnic surname was too long or unpronounceable to use. Hope his ego survived that rejection, Hartung chuckled to himself. He watched closely. Every drop of blood must be cleared from each chamber. He trusted his people, but this time his reputation at Mayo was also at stake. How easily we get caught up in our egos, he thought. Nevertheless, I wouldn't be here if I—or the team—did shabby work.

Finally, as he watched, Carolyn took the ice chest, with its precious cargo, from the OR. Hartung watched her hand it carefully to Max, who accepted it with utmost seriousness, then turned and ran off to meet the helicopter waiting on the hospital roof. Hartung thought about the little girl who would receive this organ today. This organ certainly was a jewel without price. He was glad he had treated it as such.

5:50 A.M.

Michael had called a medi-van to take him home from the hospital. Father John had offered him a ride, but his battery-operated wheelchair was far too difficult to fold and hoist into a trunk. Besides, once he was lifted out of his chair, he was helpless, with no control over his own body. He didn't like that feeling.

Also, he needed to be alone now. He'd had enough, more than enough.

The mechanics of getting the wheelchair into the van and strapped down was a good diversion to occupy his mind. The van driver, a rotund, chatty, balding man, was the same one who had brought him to the hospital. Probably he was the only one on the late night shift. Unfortunately, on the trip in, Michael had been very nervous and told the driver that his best friend had been in a serious accident.

Now, the man was anxious to pick up the conversation where it had left off. As they started moving, the questions started again. But Michael didn't want to talk to anyone—especially a virtual stranger—at a time like this.

"He died," he said—and tuned all the driver's remaining questions out of his mind.

At the handicap entrance to Michael's apartment building, the driver positioned the wheelchair onto the lift and lowered his passenger to ground level. Then he pushed Michael up the low ramp to the automatic door. Though the chair was motorized, the driver seemed to want to help, but, once inside, he seemed uncertain what to do next. Michael thanked him, expecting him to leave.

"I can take you to your apartment," the driver offered. The offer was out of the ordinary. Was it restitution for asking too many questions, Michael wondered? Or just merely human compassion?

When Michael declined his offer, the man seemed reluctant to leave. He looked at the long switchback ramp, not knowing how far Michael had to travel.

"Are you sure?"

"Yes. Thank you very much."

Once the driver closed the entrance door behind him, Michael sighed deeply, positioned his chair close to the wall, and leaned his head against the cool partition. He felt drained, lost. The long ramp extensions to the third floor loomed before him. He waited, his head braced by the wall.

I hope the battery lasts, he thought.

But, before he could begin the climb, without a signal, a gentle, blanketing sleep overtook him.

5:55 A.M.

Jan felt detached from reality, alone in the dimly lit waiting room. Nothing about this place seemed real—except that it

looked like what it was: a place where people *waited*. Like every
other waiting room she had ever seen. Not that there had been all
that many, thank God, but certainly too many recently.

Everything tonight had happened so fast. The blizzard.
She remembered that. Then the excitement in Rudy's room. She
sat back with her head against the wall and tried to remember
how it had happened. Her brain couldn't seem to capture the
craziness of that scene. She remembered thinking about the
storm. From inside, looking out, and then in a flash they were out
into that blast of cold air. The ambulance. Yes, the ambulance,
and Rudy, and Julie. It was Julie who had sustained her. Julie had
been there, and Jan knew she could trust her.

But Julie had left, deserted her among these strangers.
She felt so desperately alone. Waiting. Waiting for news. All these
weeks they had waited for this transplant. But, until now, she had
refused to think of what it entailed. She had made herself look
upon this potential cure as something innocuous. Like the
removal of an inflamed appendix, or injections of some incredible wonder drug, perhaps, that could cure his sick heart. But a
transplant. It wasn't a medicine; it wasn't simple.

Someone had died—a real person. This person had been
strong, healthy. Was it a man or a woman? She somehow had
heard, or assumed, it was a man. This person, this man, had died
to save Rudy's life. Was this the room where someone else had
waited for word of his condition? A wife? A son? A mother or
daughter?

No. She couldn't think about that now. Rudy had nothing
to do with that other death. It wasn't Rudy's fault, or hers for
that matter. It had merely *happened*. Whoever died had simply
died—in an accident probably, Julie had told her.

But what were the doctors doing right now to Rudy? To
the man who was giving his heart to Rudy tonight? She forced
herself to open her eyes. It was the only way to shut out the questions.

She looked around; the room was empty. A large, empty waiting room, and she was the only person waiting. It was so quiet. Too quiet. Only muffled sounds from behind the double doors through which she had come, and occasional clanging noises from the opposite direction. At that end of the room was a corridor that branched left and right, with a window straight across the hall from this room. She was hearing something clanking, hard, metallic—a mop handle, perhaps, hitting the side of a scrub bucket. A person walked by in that corridor, humming off key. For an instant Jan smiled, but the smile soon evaporated. She had tried to hold it longer, but a smile cannot be contained against its will.

She looked up at the acoustical ceiling tiles. Perhaps that was the one feature of all hospitals that looked the same. Jan made herself focus on the tiles. No frightening images now. She would not tolerate them.

She remembered the times she'd counted what seemed to be identical tiles as she was wheeled to the delivery room. Counting them then had taken her mind momentarily off the pain of labor. Despite the pain, those were happy times, pilgrimages of anticipation—the births of their children. Then they never doubted the outcome would be happy. The only mystery then was whether the new arrival would be a boy or a girl.

Had Rudy counted the ceiling blocks on his way to the operating room?

She wished her kids were here. No—then she would have to assure them there was nothing to worry about. She was too terrified for such bravura tonight.

Finally Macrae came through the double doors into the waiting room—the one and only familiar face Jan had seen thus far. Jan rose to her feet. What had this woman come to tell her?

"He's doing fine, Jan. He's under anesthesia, and they have him almost ready for surgery." Macrae eased herself and Jan into adjoining seats.

"Then we made it? We got him here on time?"

"Yes, indeed, you did. Not much to spare, but you made every minute he needed. Dr. Dolan asked me to tell you how sorry he was that he was unable to visit with you before the operation, but he wanted to move very quickly with Rudy's surgery. As soon as the surgery is finished, he will be out to talk with you."

Jan nodded and tried to remember Dolan's face. She only remembered the words of that last visit: no insurance, no transplant. But this was not the time for remembering such news. They had made it now. That was all that mattered.

"You had a wild trip tonight, didn't you? I don't know how you survived that frightening ride for three hours!"

Tears filled Jan's eyes. "I don't know what I'd have done if Julie hadn't come along."

"She's a real jewel." Macrae said. "I wish we could tempt her to come here to work."

Jan shook her head slowly. "But there are a lot of good people in the other hospital who need her, too."

"You're right. And speaking of good people, there are a lot here, too, who were pulling for you and Rudy to make it safely tonight." Jan could only nod.

Macrae stood up. "I just wanted to let you know that everything is proceeding beautifully. Rudy's sense of humor is intact, I can assure you. He has all the staff charmed." Those were good words to hear, Jan thought.

"And I don't suppose it will surprise you that he was worried about how you were doing."

It did not surprise her; that was Rudy. She could only smile through her tears.

Macrae checked her watch.

"He's feeling no discomfort now, and a whole team of people are monitoring every breath. When he wakes up, it will be all over. He'll be wearing his brand new heart. So you get yourself settled into a comfortable spot. There are pillows and blankets in those closets." She pointed across the room. "A reception desk volunteer will be here at seven with coffee. But, in the meantime, try to get a little rest. You've had an exhausting night."

Jan nodded continuously, too numb to separate Macrae's various assurances.

"I'll be in and out to keep you posted on each step along the way. Now, you just try to rest a little. Rudy is in very good hands."

Jan watched Macrae leave. Once she was out of sight behind the swinging doors, Jan felt the tiredness overwhelm her. Every fiber of her body sagged.

33

EARLY MORNING

6:00 A.M.

Emily McCabe followed Rudy Popovich's cart into OR
Two. It was fascinating to watch a well-trained surgical team doing
various jobs in a single flow of graceful and purposeful motion.
As an outsider observing this surgery, she was spellbound at this
undulating surge of movement. So many people, each knowing
exactly what needed to be done next to prepare a patient for what
had to be the most significant medical procedure of his life. No
wonder surgeons were so zealously loyal to their teams.

The patient had closed his eyes during most of the prep
work, but she doubted he was asleep. Most patients, she recalled,
do close their eyes when the serious procedures begin, shutting
out their feeling of exposure, nakedness—all these people staring down at one's mostly uncovered body. And many patients did
not want to know when that moment of absolute vulnerability
occurred, when sleep overtook them and they ultimately lost all
control of their individuality. It was a blessing that a patient
forgets most of this chaos when recovered from anesthesia.

She shoved herself into a corner of the operating room, hoping to become invisible.

Jonah Dolan walked into the room, his cap, mask, and shirt soaked with perspiration. Emily watched his keen eyes take in the entire scene, yet remain unfazed by the activity.

"I'm going to change and drink a gallon of water," he said to the anesthesiologist. "OR One was like a boiler." He removed his mask and moved to Rudy's side, taking his patient's hand. Rudy opened his eyes.

"Well! You created quite a bluster tonight," Dolan said. Rudy could only smile. "We're glad you could make it to our little party."

Rudy struggled to make his lips move. "My birthday party."

"Really? How appropriate to get a new heart on your birthday. May I ask how old you are today?" Of course, he'd seen the age on Rudy's chart. This was just soothing-time chatter.

Again Rudy worked to shake his head, and to speak. "No. The first day of my new life," Rudy's muttered, as tears ran down his temples. His eyes had closed, but the broad smile remained.

Jonah Dolan's voice was noticeably softer as he turned and left.

"I'll be scrubbing. Let me know when you're ready."

Emily also left—a sad-happy feeling enveloping her. She found Macrae in the middle of a corridor, in the same mood— but for different reasons.

"I think I'll wait until the actual incision on Rudy before I tell the Nicholses that this was a false alarm," Macrae said.

"Sounds reasonable," Emily responded.

"Well, it probably is reasonable. But I dread facing them—though I suspect by now they've already guessed." She headed into OR Two, where the patient was being put under anesthesia.

Emily felt suddenly extraneous. But she did want to observe this transplant procedure. Perhaps a cup of coffee would perk her up, and kill some time until Jonah was ready. She turned toward the staff lounge.

Nancy Martinez was adding milk to a cup of coffee, meaning the other kidney patient had now been transferred.

"Nancy, how good to see you again. Busy night, eh?"

Nancy laughed.

"You just spoke the two operative words of my professional life—busy and night. It's all part of the game, I guess. But at least we now have a very happy kidney recipient ready for her turn in OR. We've been very concerned about Kate Lonsdale's state of mind. But she's pulled out of her depression splendidly"

"Is she down here?"

"Nope, I put her up in a room on renal. She and her husband needed some 'catching up' conversation, and this place is crazy during transplantation. I've got her on a dialysis fix, and will start drips in about fifteen minutes. So, she'll be all ready to roll in when they're ready for her." Nancy took a sip of coffee. "Meanwhile, back to the rat race." She exited, trying to carry her cup without spilling the coffee.

6:10 A.M.

The moment the double doors swung shut behind Macrae, Jan again felt numb, empty. Almost too frightened to breathe. She tried to tell herself everything was fine. We got Rudy here on time. Dr. Anderson says this Dr. Dolan is a wonderful heart surgeon, the best. She had to trust him, but doubt lingered. Perhaps it was the memory of the last time she'd seen him, when he'd delivered his devastating news to Rudy, that left such adverse feelings. She remembered how stiff and hard his face had looked that morning. Now he had Rudy's life in his hands. She tried to forget Dr. Dolan and think about other things.

This waiting room was no help. Like everything else, it was strange to her. Feeling a chill, she tugged on her sweater. Where had she left her coat? Home? In the ambulance? It didn't matter. Nothing mattered now except Rudy. There was nothing that could warm her but the news that Rudy finally had his new heart and it was beating inside of him.

Time weighed heavily on Jan. It wasn't so much the time, perhaps, as the feeling of isolation, the crushing desperation. She waited, watching the clock tick off minutes. Why hadn't she thought to look at the clock when Macrae had gone back to the operating room? She had been staring at that large, unrelenting face all along. But she had not been registering the time. Nothing was real tonight.

A young couple came in from the corridor and sat in a corner, speaking softly to each other. The young man was crying, and his companion—his wife?—was trying to comfort him.

Jan needed someone to comfort her, someone to say, "Don't worry, Jan. It's all over now. Rudy is safe."

And she needed a bathroom. But she was afraid to leave. What if Macrae came looking for her and thought she had left?

She could wait no longer. Whatever good or bad news there was would have to wait.

"Jan, are you in here?" Macrae's voice called out.

"Yes, yes. I'll be right out."

Her hand was just reaching for the latch on the stall door. Now as she touched it, her stomach churned. Oh god, she thought! Please don't let it be bad news.

"They've started Rudy's surgery," Macrae announced. "He's doing well. He's on by-pass. A pump, a kind of artificial heart, will keep his blood circulating until the new heart is all ready for final connection."

"Oh, my," Jan said—unable to think of anything else to say. "A pump? Does that mean he's all right for now?" she asked.

Macrae nodded.

"Yes. And if all continues to go well, the pump will be working like his own heart should have been working all these years until his new heart is ready to take over the job.

And—Dr. Dolan's is very pleased with the condition of the donor heart. I saw it, too, and it's beautiful and strong. No one could ask for a better looking organ."

"Does this mean that the operation will be successful, that everything is going to be okay?"

Macrae smiled. "Well, we won't say that yet—not until the surgery is finished, and the new heart starts beating. But it looks very promising. So, hang in there. I'll be back again when there's more to report."

Jan took a deep breath and tried to relax. It's going all right, she told herself.

As she washed her hands, her gaze focused on the mirror. She hardly recognized the person facing her. Dark circles underlined her eyes, which were red and swollen from tears. If Rudy saw me like this, she thought, I'd scare him to death. A haggard smile crept onto the face in the mirror.

Rudy, she thought, you just pull through this operation and I'll put on the happiest smiling face you've ever seen. She splashed cold water on her cheeks and eyes and blotted her face dry with paper towels. She felt a little better.

When Jan returned to the waiting room, the young couple appeared to be sleeping. She found a blanket, wrapped it around herself, and settled into a chair at the opposite wall. She tried to sleep, but instead, sat waiting.

Another woman came out through the operating room doors. Jan caught a glimpse of her face and it frightened her. Was it too soon for news, she wondered? But she immediately realized the woman was not in a uniform. She was small and trim, in her late forties or early fifties perhaps, dressed very attractively in slim navy slacks, a white silky shirt, and a tweed blazer. Looking at her, Jan felt frumpy. As the woman drew closer, Jan saw that she too was fighting tears and heading to the rest room.

Jan looked at the clock again. Had the hands stopped moving? No, it was just that she had again forgotten what the time was when she last checked it. I must be losing my mind, she thought. But I guess I'm entitled. I have to do all the worrying while Rudy sleeps. The irony made her smile.

When the kids were small and she felt worried, Rudy used to make pronouncements—particularly at bed time, she remembered.

"Now Janny, you have to stop worrying. They'll come through all this just fine." Then he'd go to sleep, and in a matter of minutes he'd be snoring away as if he hadn't a care on the world. And she'd still lay awake all night worrying.

He used to tease her that he was going to hire her out as a guardian angel because she watched over him so well when he slept. And now, that's exactly what's been happening again throughout all these months of Rudy's illness, she thought. I sit and worry, and he sleeps.

It was some time before the other woman came out of the rest room. She had obviously re-done her makeup, but her eyes, like Jan's, still looked puffy and swollen.

As the woman walked by, she glanced at Jan, and their blue eyes met. Both murmured hellos, and the woman kept walking for a few feet. Then she turned back.

"Do you have someone in surgery?" She walked back and sat down near Jan.

"Yes. And you?"

"No, I guess not. My husband was an alternate for a heart transplant tonight. They haven't told us yet officially, but I'm sure it's going to someone else." She fought back tears, staring straight ahead.

Jan felt a cold knife being driven into her stomach. No words came to her lips. There was nowhere to escape to, no place to hide.

After what seemed like an eternity, the woman suddenly snapped her head toward Jan.

"It's your husband, isn't it? He's the person who's getting the heart."

Jan nodded. "I'm so sorry."

The woman looked away.

"Don't be sorry. I wouldn't have felt sorry if you'd gotten stuck out on the highway, and Jim could have this heart tonight."

Jan couldn't breathe. What was she supposed to say? Her head shook slowly from left to right, trying to deny this was happening. The woman looked at her again.

"No. That's not true. I *would* have thought about you and your husband, and I would have been sad for you—and for the family of the man who died tonight."

The moves were tentative at first, then they both reached out for each other, hugging tightly. Not until their breathing slowed did they part.

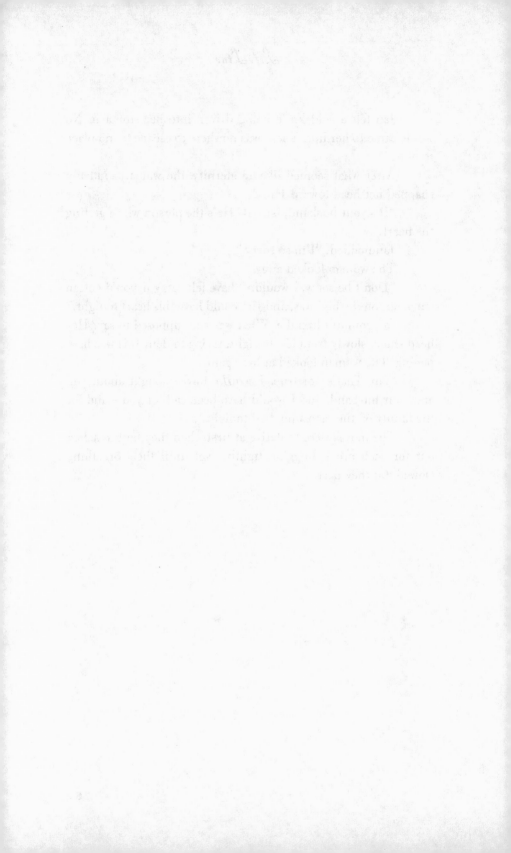

34

"AND A SMALL CHILD . . ."

6:15 A.M.

Terror was building in Alicia. This thing she and David had waited for was here. It was going to happen. These people they barely knew were going to take their beautiful child to a big, sterile operating room, put her to sleep, and cut into her precious little body. They were going to tear out a part of her and replace it with part of another person. As they drove closer and closer to Rochester, the panic built. This can't be happening, Alicia shouted silently, not to my little girl. Was this is the right thing for us to do.

David was driving too fast. Alicia wanted to tell him to slow down, but she couldn't. In the dim light reflected back off the highway, she'd seen his face and recognized the look—the grim, determined stare.

Once Patty had been put on the transplant list, Alicia had expected this particular trip to be a joyful, exciting time—getting the news, at last, that Patty would finally have a wonderful, healthy new liver. It would be the beginning of making everything good and happy again. But Alicia didn't feel good or happy—because David had asked that terrifying question.

"Could our little girl die during this operation?"

David wasn't supposed to ask that, especially not at a time like this. It was the secret dread Alicia had hidden even from herself, burying it far away from reality. But once spoken—once asked—the lethal verbalization had been brought into the open, exposing them to the deadly possibility.

As the car on the freeway turned toward Rochester, Alicia felt as if she were going to throw up. David had been lighting one cigarette from another. Alicia could barely breathe. She opened the car window a crack for fresh air.

If only he hadn't asked that question.

When he hung up the phone, she had waited in terror for the answer. But David didn't say anything. She could have asked him, but she couldn't find a way. They left without mentioning his words.

Before rousing her mother to tell her they were going to Rochester, Alicia had steeled herself with a prepared statement. In her most matter-of-fact tone she quickly said,

"The hospital called. They have a liver for Patty. We're going in now. We'll call you when we know something. You can tell the rest of the family."

She had not left time for her mother to ask questions because she didn't have any answers.

"Maybe Eddie can stay home from school today. Whatever you decide is fine."

Alicia closed the car window. She had made some instant coffee and brought it along, but she was shivering so badly she could barely sip it. David had not touched his. As the reflected glow of the city lights appeared before them, the faintest pink fleck of the new day touched over the horizon.

Finally she could wait no longer.

"Is she going to live?"

"That woman, Meg, didn't say outright. They never do. But I guess she thinks Patty will be all right," he said in an uncertain tone.

"I guess they never really know," Alicia said. Her soul felt vacant.

Walking from the elevator toward the ICU, Alicia noticed Carla, encased in an old blue sleeping bag, lying on the floor of the waiting room.

When they arrived in the ICU, Maureen greeted them, reaching out to Alicia with a hug badly needed. David went straight into Patty's cubicle, then returned to the desk.

"Any word yet?" he asked grimly.

"I'll call Meg and see if Dr. Jamison has arrived yet."

Alicia walked to Patty's bedside, leaned over, and gave her child a gentle kiss. Patty did not stir.

"Oh, my sweet baby," she whispered into Patty's ear. "You're going to come through this just fine."

Patty turned her head and opened her eyes.

"Did my new liver come yet, Mommy?"

"Yes, darling. Today you will get your wonderful transplant."

"Will it hurt?"

"You will go to sleep for a nice, long nap, sweetheart. And you won't feel anything at all. Then, when you wake up, you'll be sore where they did the operation. But you'll get medicine to make it not hurt too much. And even when it does hurt, you can tell yourself, tomorrow will be better, and the next day will be better, and each day coming. And then, before you know it, the pain will be gone, and you'll be home, playing with Eddie and your friends."

"I'll like that, Mommy." She seemed to be fading off to sleep again.

"I love you, Patty," Alicia again whispered.

"I love you, too, Mommy." The whisper was barely audible. "Is Daddy here, too?"

"I sure am, baby." David walked to the bed and leaned over to kiss her.

"Do you know that I'm getting my new liver tonight?"

"You bet I do." It was the first time Alicia had seen him smile since they had made love earlier that night.

Patty wrinkled her nose. "You smell like smoke, Daddy. Remember, you promised to stop when I got my new liver and got well again."

"Sweetheart, I'll do that and walk on a bed of hot coals for you, too."

She giggled, and her smile lingered, then slowly slipped away as she fell back into sleep.

Maureen came to the cubicle entry and whispered, "Dr. Jamison is on his way up to talk with you. Perhaps you'd like to meet him in the waiting room. We'll keep an eye on Patty."

"So you see," Dr. Jamison was explaining, "because so few child-sized cadaver livers become available, we've been helpless in the past. Now, however, we know that we can take an adult-sized organ, and trim it to fit a child's cavity. It will function perfectly, heal itself, and grow in size with the child."

Alicia has shuddered at the word cadaver. She was bewildered. This seemed so bizarre. An icy shiver ran down her back.

David's eyebrows knit together, an expression that always signaled angry confusion or disbelief. Tonight it had to be both.

"And just where did this liver come from?" he asked.

"Actually it's still on its way here—from Minneapolis."

"Who in Minneapolis?"

"A man who was killed in an accident. All the injuries were to his head. His family very generously donated his major organs for transplantation. Patty was at the top of the list for a couple of weeks, but this was the first organ that was a close enough match."

Alicia wanted to cry. This waiting room, where they had spent so many long days, now seemed so unwanting, so alien in the dark emptiness of this early morning. And now she heard that a man—the one whose liver Patty would receive—had a family. That should not have surprised her. Most people do have families. But this particular family was suffering the loss of someone they loved. Did he have to die to make Patty well?

"In a couple of hours we should have the organ here, and can begin Patty's transplant. Do you have any questions?"

Alicia felt too muddled to think of questions. Would Patty be different after getting an organ from an older man? She couldn't ask a stupid question like that, besides she knew the answer already. At least in her head, she knew. But that didn't still the nagging fears.

David finally spoke. "How long will the operation take?"

"Unfortunately, Mr. Goodwin, I can't give you a set time. It could be from eight to twelve hours. But we hope everything will go faster than that. However, let me assure you, the longer wait does not signal any problems. Patty is a small child, so the veins and arteries, as well as the cavity from the removal of her liver, will all be smaller than the donor's. So, the donor organ and the connecting tissue will have to be tailored to fit her small body. This could take some time. On the other hand, she is still a generally healthy child. That will help enormously.

"I'm sure you will be glad to know," he continued, "that Dr. Stein will be with me during surgery, along with two assisting surgeons—just to make sure we can get everything done with the maximum efficiency. Meg, your coordinator, will be in and out of the OR. So she and Dr. Stein will come out to see you periodically, to keep you informed of our progress. That should make the wait a little easier." He paused for an instant, looking at them.

"Anything else?"

They both shook their heads.

"We'll keep Maureen apprised of our readiness to start. When the attendants come to get Patty, you can go downstairs with them, and they will direct you to the waiting room."

He stood, his usually serious face tried to look upbeat, but only half succeeded. He shook their hands.

"I will see you immediately after the surgery. And I am very optimistic that we will have excellent results to report to you."

Then he was gone. And with his departure, it seemed that the room, the world, folded up and left with him.

Bleakly, Alicia sat down and stared into the dark vacuum that was trying to suffocate her.

"David, I'm terrified," she said. She looked straight ahead as she spoke. We've waited for this, but, now that it's about to happen, I'm frightened."

David sat down next to his wife and put a limp arm around her.

"I know, Alie. I know."

6:50 A.M.

Michael didn't know how long he had slept inside the entrance to his apartment house. An hour or so, perhaps, maybe more, maybe less. At the change of shifts, the night attendant, Raymond, responding to another resident's call, had discovered him. Raymond offered to accompany him up to his apartment, but Michael declined and became indignant when the man insisted on silently following behind him. However, his anger soon abated when his wheelchair stalled halfway up a ramp. He had no choice but to submit to a push.

Raymond wanted to see that Michael was safely settled into bed, but Michael did not want to change his daily routine.

Such a routine was critical, since he was dependent upon others for much of it. Most likely he would not have been able to sleep anyway. He hooked up his alternate battery and rolled himself to the window, turning off lights on the way.

Outside his window, the glimmer of the new day was creeping sluggishly across the southern sky. Infrequent snow flakes dallied in midair in the impending gray of dawn. Conditions were ripe for a blizzard.

He was grateful he was home.

Without warning, pictures of Donald infiltrated his mind: the operating room where he had had to identify his friend, the room in which he spent the silent vigil beside Donald's lifeless form, and the moment when the body—Donald's body—had been wheeled away. He would always remember the towel across Donald's face, a face that wasn't there anymore.

Abruptly, he pounded the arm of his wheelchair with what strength he has left. He willed himself to obliterate these images. He must move forward and seek out what was still alive in the world. His own life depended upon that.

Beneath the window, the streets were coming to life. Traffic began to move rapidly as a myriad of drivers propelled their cars to their jobs, hastening to arrive before the impending storm moved in. Would they get back home tonight? They might not, but still they ventured out. He'd gladly trade places with any one of them, he thought to himself.

He could see the next corner south of his apartment, but struggled to spot the one beyond that. Even without their leaves, the trees still obscured his view. He wondered which intersection was the one where Donald's accident had occurred. Had the driver been drunk? Had the police thrown him in jail? Or was it a female? No one had said, but he had envisioned the driver as a man. Did the driver have someone waiting for him—anxious, and then frantic? Was he having nightmares over what he'd done? Would he ever forget the shock he felt when he saw Donald's broken body? Did he realize the pain he had caused Margaret— and even Michael himself.

Possibly. But maybe it wasn't his fault. Donald's rattletrap bicycle had no lights. Stupid, he thought. Donny had been so hard-headed. His summer bicycle was well-equipped with front and tail lights and reflectors. He had all the safety features on a bike he used on clean streets and on nights of longer daylight. Why did his irreconcilable logic decide that his winter bike did not need them. Why didn't he use plain old common sense?

He realized the view from his window was beginning to hold him hostage. He had to derail thoughts of Donny, cut them away from the choking grip they held on his mind. He looked down at his hands, forced himself to relax, and closed his eyes. Again, sleep released him from painful, irreversible reality.

7:00 A.M.

Jan leaned her head back against the wall and tried to relax. Rudy's operation was going on at this very moment. His fate was in the hands of the doctors. Prayers were all she could lend. But she had about prayed herself out.

The other woman still sat beside her. They had both been looking at some indefinite point on the other side of the room. As a doctor approached the young couple, Jan and her new companion watched. The news was obviously bad and the young woman began to sob. A few minutes later, they left.

"I should get back," Rita Nichols said, soon afterward. "But it's so hard."

Jan understood.

"He was sleeping when I left to go to the rest room." But she remained sitting next to Jan. A smattering of new arrivals came into the room—someone new to watch. Occasionally a custodian, nurse, or misplaced visitor walked down the corridor, momentarily drawing their attention.

Their silences were lengthy and their conversation short
and to the point.

"How long has your husband been ill?"

"A couple of years."

"And yours?"

"About eight."

Other questions meandered slowly between them, each at
indefinite intervals, with corridor activity interspersed. They sat
next to one another, but neither looked at the other. Their arms
almost touched, but never quite met again since that first
embrace. After separate visits to the rest room, each felt com-
pelled to return to a seat next to the other.

Jan wished Rita would leave. Her being there made Jan
uneasy and awkward. Rita's husband was denied the heart that was
now being implanted in Rudy, and that was disconcerting. Yet, if
Rita did leave, Jan wasn't sure she could endure the isolation. She
wondered how Rita could bear to suffer being near her. Perhaps
the thought of being alone was even more frightening to face.

Finally, reality struck.

A blond nurse, dressed in hospital whites, pushed through
the surgery doors. She came to them directly. Her expression was
pleasant, but impersonal. Whom had she come to find?

"Excuse me, is one of you Mrs. Nichols?"

Rita responded, but quickly turned to Jan. Her expression
was one of panic.

"Macrae would like you to return to your husband's room
for a few minutes."

This time only Rita and Jan's hands touched. Rita's grip
sent pain through Jan's wrist. Then she and the nurse were gone.

Jan fought back her fears again. Rudy was indeed getting
another chance at life—but she already knew that. She hoped
another heart would come quickly for Rita's husband.

A gray-haired woman in a pink uniform was setting up a
coffee urn, but Jan didn't feel like coffee. Her tired, burning eyes

needed to close. She went to the wall units and found a pillow, then arranged herself on one of the little couches.

Sleep came quickly: a light, vigilant sleep.

Twice Macrae came out to report that all was going very well.

"Before long, Jan," she said on the second visit. "I should have very good news. So, just go back to sleep."

Again Jan closed her eyes. They must be getting down to the end now, she thought. Rudy was making it. Macrae had said that she'd have good news soon. She also said to go back to sleep. How on earth could Jan do that after such a message? She sat up and looked at the clock. As usual she had forgotten the time when she last checked. She wanted to call the kids, but decided against it until there was final certainty that the new heart was beating in their father. How happy and excited they would all be, she thought.

She folded her blanket, put it and the pillow on the chair next to her, then visited the rest room. The reflection in the mirror still looked worn, but different, happier. Jan combed her hair, and applied a little makeup. When she was finished, she felt reasonably satisfied with the result. I suppose one prayer answered per night should be enough, she thought. Her reflection smiled back.

7:10 A.M.

She thought she'd be able to sleep from sheer exhaustion, but she hadn't. Instead, she'd sat in an easy chair trying to stop the myriad thoughts of Donald which assailed her. Finally, Margaret forced her tired body into her nightwear. While she brushed her teeth, her face in the bathroom mirror was nearly unrecognizable. She eased herself into bed. But her body felt like a tightly-coiled spring. She could not unwind. Though she tried to close her eyes, they quickly snapped open. Even when she put her hand up to force them closed, they fought her. She needed a cup of coffee to relax herself.

Her friends always laughed when she insisted that a cup of coffee calmed her nerves. Most of them had given up caffeine years ago, in the belief that it kept them awake. But Margaret found the warm, rich liquid soothing—a gentle, pleasant tranquilizer.

This morning, it was the ritual that she found comforting—the simple rote of the preparation and the short wait as the water drained through the coffee maker. The cup's warmness in her hands seemed to bring solace to her exhausted body. She made every effort to think of nothing but the fragrant, steaming liquid. But she soon realized that she was losing the battle to block out Donald's death.

I need to arrange a funeral, she thought. There are people I must call. How can I explain about this terrible thing? Again, for a moment, she wasn't sure it had happened at all. Surely Donald would walk in the door and up the stairs to his apartment at any moment. Then reality returned.

Who should she call first? Her sister-in-law, of course. They were to be together tomorrow—or was it today? She had lost track of time. Margaret's little vacation was gone. She had wanted just a little time to be alone—not the rest of her life.

She left the phone ring until Millie answered, her voice sluggish with sleep. She sounded so far away. Margaret looked at the clock. She hadn't realized it was so late—or was it early in the morning?

"It's me," she said, hesitating for a moment.

"Margaret? Why on earth are you calling me so early? She could feel the impatience in Millie's voice.

"I can't come tomorrow."

"Well, it's already tomorrow!" Millie said, and then hesitated briefly. "Margaret, what's the matter? There's something wrong, isn't there? What's happened?"

"It's Donald." The words finally came out.

"What's wrong with him? What's he done?"

"He's dead, Millie. He's dead." Her voice cracked and disappeared, swallowed in tears.

"Oh my god! Where are you? At home?" She didn't wait for an answer. ""I'll be there in a half hour. Just stay where you are. I'll be there soon."

Numbly, Margaret returned the receiver to its cradle. She picked up her coffee cup and sipped slowly. She had taken the first step toward finalizing Donald's death. She had finally said the awful words.

"Donald is dead."

35

BUSINESS NOT AS USUAL

9:15 A.M.

John, the courier, had already gone to the helipad atop Mercy Hospital. The chopper from Minneapolis was expected momentarily. In the OR service area, Meg watched as her boss, Dr. Charles Jamison, paced the floor in front of the nursing station, pausing from time to time to look at the two baskets of charts, as if expecting some bit of data to jump out to his attention. He was suited and ready to work. So were Dr. Stein and the assisting surgeons.

Jamison finally went into the OR where Patty lay lightly anesthetized and ready for the first incision. Her small face bore a serene innocence that seemed inappropriate for what she was about to face, but he knew this was the advantage of being a child. He could only imagine the agonized expressions on her parents' faces.

The OR lights were now subdued. The first portion of Patty's preparation for surgery had been performed. For nearly an hour, Dr. Hardy, the anesthesiologist, along with three nurses, had slowly and gently been intubating intravenous lines. Then they arranged her small form on a softly padded electric blanket, which would help keep her warm during the long procedure, especially when the well-chilled liver would be laid into her body. They would take no chances on hypothermia setting in during that icy intrusion.

From the nursing station, Meg watched the nurses position the small body with great care to prevent pressure sores, or nerve damage, or too much stress on her young, fragile joints. These were always concerns for any patient during such long surgery, but particularly for the delicate body of a child. A small pillow had been placed beneath her knees, and another between her legs. Then the limbs, from the knees down, were lightly wrapped together with the pillows to avoid involuntary jerks of leg nerves. When Patty awakened, Meg thought, she would love the floppy, fleece slippers the nurses were putting on her feet. Her arms were also wrapped and slightly restrained at her sides. Finally her exposed body had been painted with Betedyne and covered to keep her warm until surgery was to begin.

Dr. Jamison stood by, scrutinizing everything, making certain that every step was perfectly executed. She wondered if he would rather have done all the work himself. Perhaps his attention to detail was merely a means of reducing his own anxiousness over this wait. He chuckled and patted the wooly slippers. Meg decided it was definitely a stress-relieving exercise. His jaw clamped rigidly again as he walked from the OR. Soon he would perform his speciality. However, there would be no opening of the patient until he had personally observed the donor organ.

Other surgeries scheduled for the day were being re-routed to other destinations. The area already swarmed with people: nurses, some re-scrubbing after the prep procedure, others waiting on stand-by; the assisting doctors and residents; hematology and respiratory technicians. An electronics specialist rested against the station desk, ready to handle any equipment malfunction throughout the long siege ahead. All of them cut a wide swath around the chief surgeon, who had resumed his pacing. He was not a man to be bumped into at a time like this.

Still others, mostly interns and residents, came stumbling through the doors in search of the *big show*. The newness of this surgery was the major draw. To each, Meg pointed upward, indicating the gallery over the OR, where authorized personnel could view techniques of different surgical procedures. It was not her responsibility to determine who was authorized. When they finally became a nuisance, she made simple, hand printed signs and taped them onto the outside of all doors to the area.

Adrienne walked in and out of the OR a half dozen times, always stopping to check the instrument tray. She had been Dr. Jamison's chief surgical nurse long before Meg had come to Mercy Hospital. Adrienne was like an extension of Jamison's arms, anticipating his call for instruments, and delivering each device in a firm, flowing movement. Watching her, Meg wondered how long it took to become that good.

Dr. Hardy remained at the head of Patty's sleeping form, an arm draped over his anaesthesia console, fingers caressing the various buttons and switches. His foot rested comfortably on the rear wheel of the surgical table. This was how anesthesiologists often positioned themselves. They were the only people who never minded standing around in the OR before surgery.

Meg checked the wall clock or her watch every few minutes. The hands never seemed to move. Between glances, she checked the desk phones, as if one of them might produce a signal that the procedure was about to begin.

She jumped when John, the courier, burst through the door, carrying the familiar Igloo ice chest. As if someone had ordered, "Battle stations!" the mass of people swarmed in different directions, hurrying toward their designated positions or lab stations.

John opened the ice chest, and Dr. Jamison removed the container. Meg followed him into the OR. He glanced upward to see the overflow crowd watching from above and nodded to them. Actually, Dr. Jamison rather enjoyed an audience. Meg had seen it before in his face. Finally, he removed the lid from the container. The liver lay, rich in color, smooth in texture.

"A perfect specimen." His voice had taken on a note of awe. "Even better than I had hoped." He looked up to his audience, who were maneuvering about for a better look at the organ. Jamison could not hear their applause, but his smile indicated he knew.

"Ms. Meghan Tyler, would you be so kind as to inform the Goodwins that we are beginning surgery."

Meg's heart pounded with excitement as she walked toward the waiting room. There was something awesome about this line of work. She couldn't have defined it, but she surely recognized it.

There is a miracle here waiting to happen, she told herself.

36

LOOKS TO THE FUTURE

9:20 A.M.

Roger was fighting sleep. He'd been trying so hard to stay awake that he'd actually become hyper-active. He couldn't relax, nor could he stay in one position for more than a few minutes at a time. He got up from the bed frequently—"to go to the bathroom," he'd told those who asked. But they had insisted on measuring his output, and, in reality, he hadn't produced a single drop. He made up all sorts of excuses for the staff who said he should be "resting." But he knew, without anyone telling him that these hours might be his last. He wasn't being morbid, just practical. And there were so many thoughts he wanted to hang onto, so many memories he wanted to linger over during this short time.

He couldn't tell anyone his reasons for remaining awake because they would begin their pep talks on the wonders of modern medicine, the surgeon's skills, and the miracle of the kidney making its way here.

Mimi, the transplant coordinator, had just popped in and

out of his room—for the twentieth time, at least—mostly cheer-leading, it seemed to Roger.

She had been there to meet him at the Emergency Room, where she introduced him to an internal medicine resident called Dr. Grange. Roger had winced. Dr. Grange, who he promptly nicknamed "Kid," looked as if he wasn't even of drinking age. Roger was in his late thirties and it disturbed him to see doctors younger than himself. He worried about their inexperience.

The "Kid" checked Roger over, the same squeezing and punching every doctor he'd ever known had done to him.

"He looks fine," the Kid reported when Mimi returned.

"Did you check his ears and his gums?"

"Ears and gums?"

"If this patient has an ear infection or some kind of gum disease, and we dose him with immunosuppressant drugs, he may well carry that infection the rest of his life, which could be rather short."

That's telling 'em, Mimi, Roger thought. He ran his tongue around his mouth, just in case. The Kid flushed, mumbled an apology, and looked into Roger's ears and mouth. All was well, the Kid reported to Mimi.

Finally Roger was taken to his room. Mimi came and went on an irregular basis, as other nurses and doctors paraded in and out, asking about his disease and its progression, and taking samples of all his fluids. He was hooked up to the dialysis machine. He grumbled loudly, realizing that he was sounding like a petulant child.

"Yes, Roger, we know you had a treatment yesterday," Mimi explained. "This is a quick fix. We want your body to be as clean as a whistle for your new kidney."

She'd been right about the short treatment, but the single hour of having to lie still had seemed an eternity. He could hear his heart racing, the sound of each beat swirling around his ears. Yet everyone who listened through a stethoscope seemed unaware that something bazaar was going on inside his body.

More blood was drawn, and new varieties of fluids added to his carcass—heavy doses of Cyclosporine and Prednisone, to encourage his system to be hospitable to the foreign organ soon to be introduced. An IV dripped clear liquid into his arm. A bag of blood hung next to the clear bag, ready to be brought on line if necessary. After all the blood they'd drawn, he was sure he needed that infusion already. Mimi did not agree when he asked her about it. Finally, when he grew drowsy, he complained that he was sure there was an additional tranquilizer or two in the drips.

Mimi accompanied yet another man into his room, and introduced the graying doctor to Roger as his surgeon, Dr. Gavin Blocker. A man in his fifties, Roger guessed. That was reassuring. But what could you tell about a man dressed in powder blue from shoe covers to his neck, except for a long lab coat covering only a portion of the suit? Nearly everyone who came in was dressed in the same uniform.

Blocker also wore a blue cap, of sorts, and had a mask hanging around his neck, which didn't quite cover his beard. Roger associated beards with men who were hiding something. He nodded and shook his head at the appropriate comments or questions that escaped from the beard. He wondered where the surgeon was that he'd met several times at the Clinic. *He* didn't have a beard.

Mimi walked out into the hall with the surgeon and they spoke briefly before she returned.

"Well, does he pass inspection? I saw you looking him over. Are you satisfied with the doctor we've selected?"

"What about that other guy I met? Do I have a choice? I'm not real strong on men with beards."

She laughed and gently shook her head at him—partly in obvious disbelief.

"Sorry, we need stronger prejudice than a beard. Beside, it's his turn on the rotation. And, while I'm at it! They tell me you're

being a tough customer," Mimi said, placing her hand on his wrist
to check his pulse. Since everyone else seemed anxious to hold his
wrist, too, he'd decided they all used that bit of stage movement as
a prop—to talk to a patient without staring down at him.

"Funny, I don't feel very tough." He fought to control the
slur in his speech. He felt like a drunk pretending to be sober.

"You've had enough sedation to drop a horse, and still you
fight to stay awake."

"Why do I have to be asleep now? I believe I'm scheduled
for a long nap this morning, aren't I?" He hoped his lips were
forming a smile. "You aren't ready for me yet, are you?"

"Not quite. Your kidney is still being maintained with the
donor, but it should be ready for takeoff before long."

"Will it be traveling by limo?"

"White Cadillac, of course. For you, nothing but the best.
And it will be nicely chilled in an Igloo ice chest."

"Any danger of someone mistaking it for a picnic lunch?"

She broke out in a peal of laughter. "I doubt it. But then
the driver might be looking for a cold beer."

Roger liked Mimi. She was funny, and yet was a take-
charge woman, a characteristic he admired in females. It was
clear from their first meeting—back when he was put on the
list—that nothing was more important to her than her patients.

A question Roger had been battling to suppress leaped to
the surface. "Do you know anything about the donor?"

"Mid to late forties. Caucasian male. Single. That's all
either of us will ever know. They did say he was very fit."

Again her face sobered.

"I finally reached your wife." Roger had been waiting for
this report—none too anxiously. He had tried to be admitted to
the hospital without telling them how to reach Martha. But Mimi
was a tough cookie. No secrets from her.

"The ringer on her phone wasn't working. The hotel's night
manager reluctantly went to her room and got her on the line."

Roger knew what was coming. Now he needed to fall asleep—instantly. He closed his eyes, but she wasn't fooled.

"She was not only shocked, but also pretty ticked off at you."

"I figured . . ." His words now seriously slurring.

"She can't get a flight out until eleven this morning. So I told her not to worry, that it was pretty obvious you didn't need her here, anyhow."

"You didn't have to tell her that."

"I know." There was a glint of mischief in her eyes; she was also merciless. "Actually, it was she who told me, Roger. And I'm telling you that if my husband pulled a stunt like this on me, I'd kill him."

"With that attitude," he said, trying to smile, "I hope you're not going to be in the operating room during my surgery."

"Oh, I'll be around. But you're lucky. I'll merely be an observer."

"Will I be out of surgery by the time Martha gets here?"

"Depends on how things go at Met General, where the donor is. Probably so. You'll be in ICU for observation, so you'll be safe from her for a day or two."

"She'll do her presentation before she leaves, won't she?" His tongue was getting thicker with each word.

"She said she didn't think she could. But I told her, if she had time, to go ahead. I assured her you'd be asleep, anyhow, and couldn't cause any more chaos around here. I think she believed me."

Now Roger really smiled. "Thanks for doing that. This presentation was important for her."

"I figured it must be important for her and for you, or you wouldn't have tried so hard to keep her from worrying." For the first time there was a softness in her voice.

Roger closed his eyes, refusing to show her how her kindness had affected him. Mimi patted his hand and started to leave.

"I nearly forgot. She said to tell you that you'd better come through this with flying colors, or she'll never speak to you again."

He tried to open his eyes and smile, but he could feel himself slipping under. He'd fought long enough. He let the soothing darkness blanket his senses.

9:30 A.M.

The Goodwins both rose quickly from their chairs when Meg entered the waiting room area. This morning it was easy enough to greet them with an encouraging smile. She saw the relief in Alicia's entire body, but Mr. Goodman maintained his grim expression.

"Good news," she said. "The donor liver arrived in beautiful condition. Dr. Jamison was very pleased with its excellent condition."

"Is Patty all right?" Mr. Goodwin seemed almost angry.

"Oh, yes. She's been in a light sleep for some time, so she could be prepared for surgery without experiencing any fear or discomfort. And the anesthesiologist, Dr. Hardy, has been monitoring her constantly since he first sedated her. He hears every beat of her heart—and those beats have been strong and regular."

"Will she be scarred?" A practical mother's question, Meg smiled to herself.

"Not really. The principal incision is from the base of the sternum," she said, illustrating on her own frame, "then curving down in an arc which follows her rib cage. Most of our patients are so proud of their new organs, and so thankful for the return of their life, that they are not bothered at all by the scar. Patty is young enough that, as she grows, the scar should become less and less noticeable."

David Goodwin's mind was still digging at something.

"This whole thing changed somehow when Dr. Jamison

said this liver was coming from a grown man. I don't know; it just doesn't seem right."

"What is it exactly that bothers you, Mr. Goodwin?"

His head rolled in frustration. "I don't know. I can't figure it out exactly. It's just that men are different from women, and grown-ups are different from kids. It just doesn't seem right mixing 'em all up."

Meg took a full breath. Now this was something new.

"There are parts of men and women, kids and adults, that are really different. Naturally below the hips is one part. And some people think we're different above the neck, too." She wished he'd caught her little witticism; but at least he seemed to be listening. "However, when it comes to mid-section anatomy, you'd be hard pressed to distinguish a male's inner mid-section from a female's. The vital organs—like the liver—are located in that middle area between the neck and the waist."

David nodded several times, slowly, thoughtfully. We're on a roll here, Meg thought. Alicia had sat back quietly, listening, and had even begun to smile.

"And that's the part of Patty that will be exchanged. No function of the liver makes us male or female, young or old—any more than a blood transfusion does."

David's expression softened. "I guess I was just afraid that my little girl would be changed by this operation, not be the same kid anymore."

"Well, she probably will be changed somewhat. For one thing she's going to be changed back to a normal, active child." That brought a real smile from this father. "And the immuno-suppressant drugs will cause some rounding of her face and more body hair, especially at her eyebrows.

"And there might be other more subtle changes. Most adults, and many children, who have been through these terrible illnesses and the traumatic wait for a transplant organ, do come out of transplantation changed. There's no way to predict those changes. Some adults become more religious; others feel real joy at each day they live. A few think they are invincible, and become quite reckless. Some time ago, one of our young adult recipients died when he drove his car at an unbelievable speed and caused a driving accident. He snuffed out three other lives, along with his own."

"I'll be damned," David said, shaking his head in disbelief.

"How about children?" Alicia asked.

"I don't think I can be very specific—age, home and school background make such differences in children. Some, as you may have guessed, leave the hospital rather spoiled and demanding after weeks or months of special attention. Mothers often say they have to wean them back into the family routine and acceptable behaviors again." Alicia smiled and nodded. "Some become overly concerned about their health—which, by the way, is another problem with some adults.

"Fortunately, Patty's disease has moved very quickly, and her return to health should also be quite rapid. Children Patty's age usually adjust quite nicely. And they are even more likely than adults to look back upon this whole experience as 'no big deal.' However, there is one downside. Children are more likely to feel annoyance or even depression at having to take their medications afterwards. That may, at times, be a hassle for Patty and for you. You'll have to monitor her closely. But if that becomes a concern for you, we can always provide professional help through our social workers or a psychologist."

David Goodwin looked at Alicia. "My questions probably sounded crazy."

"No, not at all," Meg insisted. "They sounded like the concerns of a loving father. And now, I better get back and find out for you what is going on in the OR."

Mr. Goodwin rose and put out his hand. "Thank you, Meg."

"You're most welcome, David."

"From me, too" Alicia added.

Meg smiled at them both and left.

9:45 A.M.

Jan walked into the corridor and looked out the window. Through the tinted glass the clouds looked pinkish-brown to the east, but darker brown to the west. Snow? Perhaps. It didn't matter now. By drawing her point of vision inward to the glass surface, she saw the mirrored image of the well-lit waiting room behind her. She felt a smile rush through her. It's too soon to know for sure, she told herself, and tried to keep the level of excitement down by refocusing on the world outside.

As she watched the front entrance of the hospital, off to the side, she speculated on people coming into the building. Were they visitors? It was certainly early in the day for mere social visits—unless a loved one was very ill. Some carried flowers or gift-wrapped packages. That was nice.

A sleek, dark limousine pulled up to the curb. The driver stepped out and opened the back door for a woman wearing a long, full mink coat. The driver moved quickly to remove an expensive-looking suitcase from the trunk and handed it to his passenger. Perhaps she was bringing clothing to her husband— but not in such beautiful, flowery luggage. This was a feminine bag. The woman spoke to the driver, who removed his cap as they exchanged a brief communication. Then they shook hands, and she turned and walked slowly toward the entrance, She paused ever-so-briefly before opening the door. Jan tried to read her facial expression. Was it pain, or fear, or despair that she saw? Jan felt sad for her. Some problems can't be cured with money, she thought.

A few snow flakes lingered outside the window before melting. More were surely coming. Soon, Rudy and she would be back home in front of the fireplace, watching the snow build its magical sculptures. Inside herself, she felt the ache that had begun when Rudy became ill begin to seep out of her body. Suddenly, she saw Macrae's reflection through the surgery area doors and turned. Macrae came toward her with a beaming smile on her face.

Joyful tears slid from Jan's eyes.

37

A MUTUAL LOVE AFFAIR

9:50 A.M.

Patty's surgery began uneventfully. Dr. Jamison's ranking associate, Dr. Cook, did the opening. This was not unusual, Meg had learned during her apprenticeship in the transplant program. However, it happened more often when Dr. Jamison was scheduled for two or more major cases in one day. Attending surgeons commonly did the preparatory opening on each patient assigned to Dr. Jamison's roster, then the chief moved in for the critical stages, with others closing the patients when the "star" was finished. That was common practice for widely-recognized surgeons, whose schedules were loaded with patients who needed or wanted the expertise that accompanied the reputation.

This morning, as others prepared for the removal of the diseased liver, Jamison seemed totally preoccupied with scrutinizing the fine, new donor organ.

Meg stood, as she usually did, at the periphery of the surgical team. Everyone was quiet as Patty's non-functioning liver was lifted from its cavity. Dr. Jamison turned, then stared, seemingly stunned as he gazed at the pale, hard organ.

"You'll send that specimen to pathology?" he asked Dr. Cook, who was already placing it on a lab dish.

"Oh yes. Let's hope it tells us something about what happened to this poor little girl."

Dr. Jamison returned his attention to the small table where the stainless steel container embracing the prized replacement organ lay. Meg slowly edged her way around the circle of surgical staff to within three feet of him. She watched with fascination. He seemed completely absorbed with this perfectly formed specimen, almost as if it were the first human liver he had ever seen. He lifted one side, then another, peeking underneath. He was so transfixed that he seemed not to notice Meg's presence. Suddenly, he looked up at her.

"All right, Meghan!" She had never seen him so elated. "It's time to get to work, isn't it?"

10:30 A.M.

The waiting room was nearly full. At Alicia's suggestion, David had gone out for a cigarette. She wished he wouldn't smoke, because of the health risks. However, when he needed a cigarette, he was like a caged animal; so, for now, it was best to let him go. She wondered if he would honor his promise to Patty to stop smoking. He adored her and it might just turn the trick. Alicia fervently hoped so.

When David returned and sat down beside her, he seemed momentarily more relaxed, but at intervals he stood up and paced back and forth—sometimes into the hallway or around the crowded waiting room, looking increasingly agitated. When he sat again, he turned partially away from her, staring off into space in that aloof way she hated.

Alicia's inner turmoil festered. She could no longer contain her tears. Unable to speak or to control the fear and the anger building inside her, she sobbed, unleashing volcanos of hot tears that flushed out secluded agonies she had barely recognized herself. Finally, she exploded.

"I hate that stoic facade you wear when I need your love and compassion so desperately."

David turned to her, looking helpless and confused. He leaned over to put his arm around her, but she lashed out at the arm with her fists, then rose and ran out to the corridor. David followed, and again tried to take her in his arms, but she fought him off. Her fists flayed against him and then fell limp against his chest. Suddenly he took her into his arms, holding her so tightly she could scarcely breath. Yet she did not want him to let go.

"Oh, Alie, I've been a fool. Some idiot notion in my head said I had to be strong, not show fear, not let go for even a minute." He loosened his grip, but still held her.

"I was supposed to be the protector in this family—for you and Patty, and Eddie, too. But I failed. I'm the man, and I'm supposed to hold it all together. I failed at that, also. I was so afraid that if I ever let go, if I ever let down my guard and showed any sign of weakening at all, I'd crack to pieces."

"But you've been so withdrawn, and then so angry."

"Not angry at you, Alie. Honest. Angry at this devilish sickness of Patty's; angry that I couldn't fix it; and angry at myself because I wasn't able to give you what I knew you needed."

"But, don't you see?" she asked. "Your silence terrified me. I felt your inner rage was directed at me, as if you held me responsible for Patty's illness."

"Oh, Alie, how could you ever think that?"

"Maybe because I was fighting so hard and so unsuccessfully not to blame myself. It seemed logical to me that you also blamed me. Then last night when you made love to me and told me you loved me, I thought the blame was finally past, that now neither of us believed this illness was anyone's fault. I was so enormously relieved, and that was why I cried. It had been so long since I had felt free of the guilt, and still loved.

"But then, after the phone call, you turned yourself back off again. You didn't say a word to me. I knew what was going to happen only from hearing your end of the phone conversation. I felt ignored, used, as if you had been playing a rotten game with me. Get what you need, then to hell with Alicia. And then I thought about what was going to happen to my poor baby's little body, and I had to accept my own condemnation again."

"Alicia, our love last night was no game. You have to believe me. It was incredible to feel joy again, even for just a little while. But when that call came, I panicked all over again. And, when I heard about the donor, what should have been good news suddenly became so horrifying, so unnatural. I don't know, Alie, I guess I just went crazy again with the guilt and the fear."

"Oh, David, how could I know?" Her arms stretched up over his shoulders. "How can either of us know what the other is feeling if we don't dare talk about bad things? As long as we can talk to each other, as long as we can share the fears and pain together, we'll be all right. I know that we can face whatever comes."

"Whatever comes," he said, once again holding her as if their lives depended upon that grasp.

11:00 A.M.

Dr. Smith crossed the busy waiting room. Alicia saw him from the corridor, and she and David hurried to meet him. His large, comfortable hands, reached for theirs.

"Please, please, let's sit down." Two chairs were open nearby, and the physician drew up another directly in front of them.

"Our little princess is sleeping comfortably," he smiled brightly. "And they're all working feverishly to complete this transplant."

"How can we ever thank you, doctor," David said. "We know she's in good hands as long as you're over-seeing that army."

"You know," Alicia said, "she thinks you rank second only to Santa Claus as the greatest person on the face of the earth." Smith smiled.

"Well, it's certainly a mutual love affair." His face sobered slightly. "I believe Dr. Jamison told you that he was trimming the donor organ. They nodded.

"But don't worry; it will soon be a perfect fit for her small body." His optimism restored their confidence.

When Smith finally parted the sea of people to return to the operating area, Alicia and David waited once again. But this time they shared the dream of a future for their child.

38

KATE

Kate Lonsdale was awake. At least she assumed so, though opening her eyes took more effort than she could summon.

She tried to separate her lips, but they were stuck together. There seemed to be a piece of flannel in her mouth. No, that was her tongue, but it was so dry she could hardly make it move. She felt cold, terribly cold.

Pain attacked her right side. Had her appendix been removed? No, that happened long ago. But maybe this was long ago, and she was just awakening from that surgery.

Something tight choked her arm. A blood pressure cuff. A voice, hollow and far away, came into her semiconsciousness.

"Katherine?" Someone was calling her, but where was she?

"Katherine, are you awake?"

Cold, she tried to call out, but they couldn't hear her. I'm so cold, she thought.

She struggled again to open her mouth. It opened only a slit for air to pass through. She felt something cool and wet, like lemon, on a stick, gently separating her lips.

"Katherine, can you open your eyes for me?" For whom? Why should I open my eyes for someone I don't know? But she tried, and they opened slightly. But the pupils quickly slipped back under the top lids, and she could see nothing. The wielder of the lemon stick swabbed out Kate's mouth. It felt and tasted fresh.

"That's the way. Now look back down at me." Who was she supposed to see?

When her eyes finally focused, a short, red-haired woman in white, barely taller than the side rails of the bed, stood next to the bed.

"Cold," Kate said.

"Well, we can do something about that; just hang on and I'll get another blanket from the warmer." Katherine fought sleep; she wanted to feel that warm blanket.

"Here we are," the nurse said as she replaced one blanket with another. It felt warm against her body, but did nothing for the inside coldness.

"Your body is chilled from your transplanted kidney," the nurse explained. "The sooner you begin to move a little, the quicker you'll feel warmer."

Her eyes slid shut again.

"Katherine. Come on, dear, open your eyes."

It took so much effort.

"Side hurts."

"Yes, Katherine, that's where your new kidney is implanted."

She remembered that. Someone had told her before surgery that they would transplant the kidney down in the area of her appendectomy scar.

"Hurts," she repeated.

"I know it does." The voice sounded sincere. "But we can't start pain medication until you're fully awake." That wasn't fair. Why did she have to be awake, only to be put back to sleep?

"Bobby?"

"Your husband and your parents are out in the waiting room. They can visit you when you get to ICU."

She faded in and out of sleep as she was moved through a pair of open doors, through an area of softer lights, then back into brightness again. She heard her own voice cry out from the stab of pain as she was moved from cart to bed.

"It's all right now, Katherine." Another voice.

"I'm giving you something for pain." Kate felt the pressure of the needle, but not the prick; there was too much pain inside.

The medication quickly sent a trail of warmth through her body.

"Would you like me to bring your husband now?"

She hoped she was nodding yes. But when the nurse left, Kate drifted back to sleep.

Bob was at her side when she awoke. His smile said it all. She had made it.

"I love you, Katie." She hoped she was nodding.

Bob took her fingers in his warm hands and kissed them. Now his warmth spread.

"You parents are here, sweetheart," Bob said. "I think we're going to be fine from now on. We've learned to understand each other a lot better in just this time we've been waiting together. I believe Kathleen has already taught me a lot about the feelings of a parent."

His hand followed hers to his face; she touched his lips, and he kissed her fingers.

"I was afraid of losing you, Bobby, losing everyone."

"We were all afraid. But now the doctor says you've come through beautifully, and you'll be home in ten days."

"Ten days!" That was so long. "What about Kathleen?"

"We're bringing her home tomorrow—your parents and I.

I've still got nurses scheduled, but I'm not sure your mother will endure them for very long. Is it all right with you if she earns her grandmother stripes until you get home."

"She'll have Kathleen spoiled rotten, even in ten days." She felt her whole face smiling. "But I guess we can turn her back into a normal child again after Mom leaves."

"Good decision, because if you didn't agree, you would have had to break the news to your mother." She smiled at him. She was sure.

"Anyhow, you'll be in ICU for a couple of days, and then you'll have a private room. Your mother is already planning sneaky ways to slip Kathleen in to visit her mommy. I know your parents want to see you. Are you up to it?"

"Oh, yes, darling. But you'll come back, won't you?"

"Nothing can keep me away."

"Oh. No one told me. Where did my kidney come from?"

"All I was told is that it came from a man who was killed in an accident. Never married, few relatives."

"How sad," Kate said.

"Remember, Kate, you were not responsible for his death. He died, and his family wanted part of him to live on. So, that's your responsibility now—to live a rich, full life for him and for us and our baby." He kissed her again, and turned to leave.

As she watched Bob walk away, Kate smiled. How good it was to be alive, devising schemes, making plans, thinking of the future.

1:30 P.M.

Roger Burrows opened his eyes and saw her.

"You son-of-a-bitch! Why didn't you tell me?" she asked.

"Martha," he said. "I'm really sorry."

"Oh, my darling, I love you so much." She cried.

"Same here." He smiled.

"Is there anything you need?" She stopped crying.

"Later, sweet woman. Doc says maybe a month." Still he smiled.

"Why, you lecherous man!"

They both smiled. Then he slipped back into a happy sleep.

39

DAY'S END

7:00 P.M.

In spite of a plodding fatigue, Meg had been determined to make it through to the end—her first "solo" as a transplant coordinator. This was too great an occasion for her to miss any part of it. As the day moved on into January's early darkness, Dr. Stein, who also had insisted upon staying on, continued to escort her when she took news to the waiting family.

During her many trips to the waiting room, Meg had seen the congregation of faces change. There had been a complete rotation of people between her visits. Only Alicia and David remained constant.

Now, they sat at the far end of the waiting area, looking contented. As she and Dr. Stein approached, the couple stood, a sudden nervous expectancy carved onto their faces.

"It's over," Meg said, happy to announce such joyful news at last. A short burst of excitement followed, then quickly hushed as all eyes went to the doctor.

"And it went superbly," Dr. Stein added.

Both David and Alicia began to cry happy tears. Meg hugged them both. Dr. Stein followed suit.

Smiles bloomed everywhere.

"Well, Meg and I must get back to check our little patient, but I know Dr. Jamison will be out shortly."

After slapping some water on his face and combing his hair, Dr. Jamison went out to see the Goodwins, reporting that Patty was doing beautifully and had been moved to ICU. They would be able to see her shortly, for a few minutes. Meg followed him out to the waiting room, but she remained some distance behind him and off to the side, not wanting to take anything away from his grand moment. However, they found themselves in the midst of a lusty gala, spotlighted by the blazing beacons of the media. For a moment, Meg wondered who had tipped the reporters off, then realized that, in a small city like Rochester, where medicine is a major industry, medical news is always heralded. She recognized several doctors and a number of residents, who had also joined the throng—and the applause. The star bowed humbly to the ovation. Dr. Jamison was grandly within his element—a most deserving honoree.

Meg watched him smile at his admirers, obviously enjoying their adulation, while answering the media questions with a modest flair. She slipped away, knowing no one would miss her. She felt overwhelmed as she left the happy group.

"I was part of something splendid today," she said quietly to herself.

40

DONALD'S LOVED ONES

Margaret and Michael's friend, Father John, officiated at Donald's funeral service, the Mass of Resurrection.

Father John placed his hand on Donald's coffin.

"I realize," he told the assembled few, "that Donald would *not* have wanted to be here with us this morning." A smile crossed every face.

"But I think he would understand how much *we* need *him* to be with us for this occasion.

"Today we seek comfort in Jesus' promise: 'Blessed are the peacemakers, for they shall be called the children of God.' And this was Donald: a peacemaker. Surely he has been called to the Father as one of His own."

He spoke of the younger Donald, idealistic and filled with unattainable dreams of peace for the world

"Over the years," he continued, "Donald seemed to be at war with the world that he believed rejected his dream. And the world was the poorer for not having known this gifted man. But

Donald did share with a rare few the magnitude of his brilliant mind, and they are the better for his intelligence and for his companionship."

Margaret and Michael smiled at one another.

"Also over those years, Donald wanted to believe that he was at war with God. But God would neither fight with, nor let go of Donald. And in the days just before his untimely death, Donald was unwittingly drawn to a reawakening of his relationship with a loving God.

"Today we draw comfort from knowing that Donald is at home with his loving Father—and that still part of him lives. For in his death he has bequeathed new lives to four grateful families whose loved ones have been recipients of Donald's transplanted organs.

"Those families know the enormity of his gift. And they—like ourselves—will never forget this rarest of men.

"Greater love than this hath no man than that he lay down his life for another."

Epilogue

THE FOLLOWING DECEMBER

The cold, cloudy day foretold snow to come. Margaret hoped to get all her Christmas errands done before more snow and ice kept her home-bound again.

She pulled her car up to the curb across the street from the apartment house. The street was one-way, and it was easier for her to get out of the car onto the road surface than to struggle with snow banks. She took time to appreciate the Christmas decorations in the windows of the apartment building. Margaret knew she was stalling, not certain she was prepared to see Michael again—to possibly relive the pain of Donald's death.

A small group of young men, mostly in wheel chairs, were gathered outside the building entrance, smoking. One, not encumbered, walked across the street to Margaret's side as she struggled to put on her coat and climb out of the car. He was young, in his twenties, with light blond hair. She thanked him as he helped her across the street and directed her to the front elevator in the building.

On the third floor landing, Michael was waiting. For a brief interlude they held hands, fighting the tears, saying nothing.

Seeing one another again, even after eleven months, ruptured still thinly healed wounds. Then, their hands separated and each took a fresh, deep breath.

They talked about banalities as they moved toward the back of the building where Michael had his apartment. Did she have trouble finding the building? Gracious, it certainly is cold and raw today. Yes, she feels very lucky to still be driving, even if only around her home area. How long has he lived here? She remembers the old houses that were once on this property. Yes, she had found someone to shovel her out after it snowed.

Finally, they were in his apartment. Very neat and clean, she noted. And orderly—except for some small watercolor paintings, most no larger than a sheet of typing paper, scattered about. The walls were full of pictures and several tables had small stacks of drawings piled on them.

Why had Donald never mentioned Michael was an artist?

"These are beautiful," she remarked. She strained her eyes to see the small initials on the corner of one of the paintings. Yes, these are Michael's, she thought. All of them!

Michael had remained silent until she turned back to him.

"He never told me!" She blurted out.

Michael smiled.

"I have a feeling there are a lot of things we've never heard about each other." He indicated a chair.

Still standing, she removed a decorated tin from a plastic grocery bag and handed it to Michael.

"I still enjoy making Christmas cookies," she said, apologetically.

"Now that was something he *did* tell me about."

They both laughed, relieving the tension between them.

She sat down, and, for a brief moment, they were silent. Then Margaret opened her purse.

"This is the letter I told you about over the phone," she said. "I thought you might like to see it."

"Do you know who it's from?"

"No. The LifeLine people say they can't tell me.

"Can't—or won't?"

"Won't—I guess. They say it has to be this way. Something about confidentiality. I have a vague recollection of hearing about it," she paused. "That night." She shuddered briefly, lost in remembrance.

"Yes, I recall that, too," Michael replied. "I think the woman who talked to us mentioned it. And, before she came, I had asked the doctor who would get the organs if you signed. He said he didn't know yet. The selection would be done by a computer. And, even after that, he said we would never know."

They lapsed into silence again until Margaret realized the envelope was still in her hand. She handed it to Michael and he looked at it.

"This came from the procurement agency."

"Yes. I guess that's the way they handle it."

Slowly, Michael carefully removed the paper from the envelope, unfolded it, and looked back at Margaret, seeming to ask for her permission to read it.

"Would you read it aloud?" She asked. "I started to read it at home and I had to stop. My eyesight is getting bad, I think. I probably need new glasses." She knew it was a feeble lie, and, from his expression, she saw that he knew, too. Silly, she thought, not wanting the depth of her still raw emotions to be known.

Michael nodded and looked back at the unfolded paper and its neat penmanship.

"To the family of donor 1126:

I can't begin to tell you the elation we felt on the night of January fifteenth when the call came. We think we have a heart for you.

I was hospitalized at the time and was rushed by ambulance to Minneapolis—it being too stormy for the helicopter.

Our only unhappy thought at the time was that in order for us to have this tremendous opportunity, someone had to lose a loved one.

I am married and the father of nine children. I live in rural Duluth and enjoy trapshooting, bowling, and hunting. I am now able to participate in these activities again, but before I was on the verge of death, having had the heart disease for eight years. But my condition had deteriorated rapidly in the last few months.

I cannot begin to thank you, the donor's family, adequately. Nothing can say what it means to be able to continue life with my family.

Thank you again.
Recipient 1126"

Michael had paused several times while reading the letter. He was obviously having trouble with his eyesight, too. Now he was silent. He sat, still looking at the letter. Rereading it, Margaret thought.

"This was a good thing we did, wasn't it?" she asked, nodding her head as if for self-assurance.

"A very good thing," he repeated. "And it is what Donny would have wanted, too."

His voice trailed off, and he shook his head slowly. He folded the letter, slid it back into the envelope, smoothed it and extended it toward Margaret.

As she reached for it, she met his glance.

"Donald's life was not wasted," she said, with a steady assurance.

Michael handed her the envelope and spoke softly but firmly.

"Nor was his death."